BARNES & NOBLE HEALTH BASICS™

IBS

By Debra Gordon

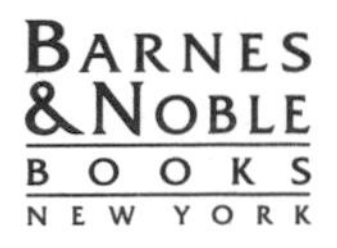

ISBN 0760756112

First Edition
Printed and bound in the United States of America

Barnes & Noble Publishing, Inc.
122 Fifth Avenue
New York, NY 10011

About the Author

Debra Gordon is an award-winning journalist who has been writing about health and health care for more than 15 years. Her work has appeared in *Family Circle, Better Homes and Gardens, Good Housekeeping, Reader's Digest*, and *Diabetes Today*. She lives in northeastern Pennsylvania, where she is a full-time freelance writer specializing in health and medicine. She is the author or co-author of the consumer health books *Cut Your Cholesterol!*, *Asthma and Allergy Relief, Eat to Beat High Blood Pressure*, *7 Nights to a Perfect Night's Sleep*, and *Maximum Food Power for Women.*

About the Contributors

Portions of this work were reviewed by Stephen Possick, M.D., and Anna Longacre, M.D. The information on mediation and biofeedback was provided by Lawrence Edwards, Ph.D.

Barbara J. Morgan Publisher
Barnes & Noble Health Basics™

Barb Chintz Editorial Director
Leonard Vigliarolo Art Director
Gina Graham Editorial Assistant
Della R. Mancuso Production Manager

Medical Illustrations by Cynthia Saniewski

Table of Contents

Foreword 6

Chapter 1 Getting the Diagnosis 7–26
Experiencing the symptoms **8** Testing for IBS **10** Similarities to other illnesses **12** Similarities cont'd **14** Getting a diagnosis **16** Types of IBS **18** Why me, why now? **20** The big picture **22** Keeping a health journal **24** Helpful resources **26**

Chapter 2 How IBS Affects Your Body 27–40
Everyday digestion at work **28** Your stomach at work **30** Your bowels at work **32** Why diarrhea happens **34** Why constipation happens **36** Why gas and bloating happen **38** Helpful resources **40**

Chapter 3 Your Support Team 41–62
Creating a health team **42** Your primary care doctor **44** Your gastroenterologist **46** Your pharmacist **48** Your dietitian **50** Working with a therapist **52** Your advocate **54** Using your health journal **56** How to be a smart patient **58** Joining a support group **60** Helpful resources **62**

Chapter 4 Treatments for IBS 63–82
Your treatment plan **64** The elimination diet **66** Over-the-counter relief **68** Probiotics **70** The brain/gut connection **72** Prescriptions for symptom relief **74** Cutting-edge drugs for IBS **76** Sleep medications **78** Psychological therapy **80** Helpful resources **82**

Chapter 5 Overlapping Syndromes 83–94
Fibromyalgia **84** Chronic fatigue syndrome **86** Interstitial cystitis **88** Migraine **90** Chronic pelvic pain **92** Helpful resources **94**

Chapter 6 The Role of Nutrition and Exercise 95–116
Food fundamentals **96** A food diary **98** Fiber and IBS **100** The fructose question **102** The role of fat in IBS **104** Food intolerances **106** What about alcohol? **108** Reading food labels **110** Eating right **112** Exercise and IBS **114** Helpful resources **116**

Chapter 7 Women and IBS 117–128
IBS and menstruation **118** Zelnorm and Lotronex **120** Pain and women **122** Pregnancy and IBS **124** IBS in women vs. men **126** Helpful resources **128**

Chapter 8 Children and IBS 129–138
What the doctor needs to know **130** Diagnosing IBS **132** A personal treatment plan **134** Stress in children **136** Helpful resources **138**

Chapter 9 Using the Internet 139–154
Evaluating Web sites **140** Top IBS health sites for consumers **142** Top medical sites on IBS **144** Researching doctors **146** Alternative approaches **148** Online support **150** Newsgroups **152** Helpful resources **154**

Chapter 10 Stress and IBS 155–172
What is stress? **156** Chronic stress and IBS **158** Assault on mind and body **160** Smart IBS coping strategies **162** Take an IBS stress inventory **164** Learning to relax **166** Your partner's concerns **168** On the job **170** Helpful resources **172**

Chapter 11 Complementary Therapies 173–192
What to expect **174** The complementary approach **176** IBS and stress management **178** Biofeedback **180** Meditation **182** Herbs, vitamins, and minerals **184** Hypnotherapy **186** Acupuncture **188** Yoga, the "mindful" exercise **190** Helpful resources **192**

Chapter 12 The New Normal 193–206
Life with IBS **194** Stages of adjustment **196** Beyond acceptance **198** Beginning the journey **200** Talking about it **202** Creating a new life **204** Helpful resources **206**

Glossary 207
Index 216

Foreword

If you are the one in five Americans with Irritable Bowel Syndrome, known as IBS, then you know how hard it is to live with IBS, let alone to get a correct diagnosis of it. Chances are you don't even know when or how your IBS started. It may have come on after a bout of the flu or a bad meal or a particularly rough patch at school or work. While some research shows that certain things can trigger IBS, no one knows why or how it continues. It doesn't help that many people still consider IBS a stress problem—or even a symptom of the imagination. It is ever so much more than that. IBS is a medical disorder that, to date, has no known cause, but has a wide array of symptoms unpredictable in both their timing and their severity. The good news is that thanks to new research that you will find here inside *Barnes & Noble Health Basics: IBS*, doctors now have clear criteria to use when making a diagnosis of IBS. And while research into the cause of IBS continues, exciting new research on the brain/gut connection has brought forth new treatments that have helped many with IBS to better manage their symptoms.

There is much you can do to feel better. You can start right here with *Barnes & Noble Health Basics: IBS*, where you'll find expert guidance from leading physicians who help you make sense of your symptoms and the various treatments available. There is also vital information on diet and nutrition, as well as tips on putting your health team together, and smart advice for stress relief.

With all these helpful insights at your fingertips, you'll be able to take control of your IBS and become an advocate for your health. It all comes down to this: An informed patient is an empowered one. So read on to put yourself in the driver's seat when it comes to your IBS.

Barb Chintz
Editorial Director
Barnes & Noble Health Basics Series

Chapter 1

Getting the Diagnosis

Experiencing the symptoms 8

Testing for IBS 10

Similarities to other illnesses 12

Similarities cont'd 14

Getting a diagnosis 16

Types of IBS 18

Why me, why now? 20

The big picture 22

Keeping a health journal 24

Helpful resources 26

Experiencing the symptoms
what's going on?

At first, you blame your stomach cramps on what you had for dinner. The cramps abate, but you now have diarrhea. It lasts for a few days and then stops. You are pretty sure it was just a stomach bug—until it happens again the following week. This time you notice that your diarrhea is followed by constipation. After a few days you are back to normal, only to go through the same cycle a few weeks later. Chances are you are also feeling a bit fatigued and depressed. You can't tell whether your problem is your stomach or your bowel or both. Are you allergic to some sort of food? Do you have an ulcer? A parasite? What is the problem? You try over-the-counter remedies to help with your symptoms. But if this strange pattern of pain continues, it's time to make an appointment to see your doctor.

Most likely your doctor will start your exam by asking you about the specifics of your plight. When did your trouble start? Where is the pain? What does your stool normally look like? How many times a day do you have a bowel movement? How long does the diarrhea or constipation last? Is there mucus in your stool? Do you have symptoms such as nausea, vomiting, or weight loss? Your answers to these questions are vital. The problem is that most people don't pay the right kind of attention to their bodies, so they don't know how to talk effectively to their doctors about their symptoms—which is doubly so if the symptoms involve problems with digestion and bowel movements. Some people are so embarrassed that they do not even go to the doctor for help, and if they do, they do not provide useful information that would help a doctor better understand their problem.

What can you do about this all-too-common communication gap between doctor and patient? For starters, you need to know what symptoms typically arise with the disorder known as **irritable bowel syndrome**, or IBS. This is especially important because while this syndrome has been around for ages, the name IBS has only entered the medical lexicon in the late 1990s when a group of doctors set the criteria for its diagnosis. Having any of the following symptoms does not mean that you have IBS, but it does mean that you need to see a doctor who is familiar with this particular disorder.

Common Symptoms of Irritable Bowel Syndrome

- Abdominal pain or discomfort usually associated with bowel movement.
- Recurrent diarrhea. An often urgent need to move your bowels comes on, resulting in frequent, loose, often watery bowel movement.
- Recurrent constipation. Often alternates with diarrhea. May be hard, difficult-to-pass stools, or unusually infrequent bowel movements.
- Abnormal stool frequency (may be defined as greater than three bowel movements per day or less than three bowel movements per week)
- Abnormal stool passage (straining, urgency, or feeling of incomplete evacuation)
- A bloated feeling
- Flatulence (gas)
- Mucus in the stool
- Chronic fatigue

Red Flags for Bowel Symptoms

If you experience any of these symptoms, call your doctor immediately:

- Sudden high fever
- Weight loss
- Blood in stools
- Pain in the gut that awakens you from sleep or interferes with sleep

Testing for IBS

diagnostic tests and X-rays

Chances are you will see more than one doctor before you get a correct diagnosis of IBS. In fact, it typically takes four years from the onset of symptoms to get a correct diagnosis of IBS. If your symptoms are not abating, it is important that you see a doctor familiar with gastrointestinal disorders (see pages 46–47 for more). There are many diagnostic tests you may need to take, depending on the severity and duration of your symptoms. Here are the range of tests.

Blood tests. These tests can screen for anemia and thyroid disorders whose symptoms can often mimic IBS. They will also test blood electrolytes, including calcium and potassium.

Celiac sprue tests. This set of blood tests looks for antibodies that indicate the presence of celiac disease, which is caused by a food allergy to gluten (found in wheat).

Erythrocyte sedimentation rate. This one-hour blood test measures the rate (in millimeters per hour) at which red blood cells settle in unclotted blood in a specially marked test tube. Elevated sedimentation rates may be helpful in ruling out an inflammatory disease, such as rheumatic arthritis, certain cancers, and/or inflammatory bowel disease, such as Crohn's disease.

Lactose intolerance tests. These tests determine if you are missing the enzyme called **lactose** needed to digest a sugar found in dairy products. After fasting overnight, you drink a flavored liquid that contains lactose. Your doctor then measures your exhaled breath for levels of hydrogen, a byproduct of the bacteria that break down the lactose that is not absorbed, or tests your blood for levels of glucose, another product of lactose breakdown. You may be lactose intolerant but not have IBS.

Physical exams:

Pelvic examination. This examination, performed on women, is conducted to rule out ovarian tumors, cysts, and other pelvic disorders that can have symptoms similar to those of IBS.

Endoscopy. This test uses a thin flexible tube that is inserted down the throat and into the stomach. At the end of the tube is a tiny camera and light that allows the doctor to view the lining of the esophagus and stomach.

Sigmoidoscopy or **colonoscopy.** These tests involve viewing the **colon** and other parts of the digestive system through a flexible tube inserted through the **anus**. The flexible sigmoidoscope views the **rectum** and **sigmoid colon** via a flexible tube with a camera and light on the end. The colonoscopy views the entire colon and usually requires anesthesia. Note: IBS-like symptoms and a family history of colon cancer or inflammatory bowel disease will most likely require a colonoscopy, especially if you are over age 50.

Stool tests. These tests check your fecal matter, or stool, for any signs of parasites or blood.

Body imaging tests:

Upper and lower GI series. To measure the size of the intestines and bowel and see if there are any lesions or ulcers, you may be given barium, either to drink for an upper GI or by enema for lower GI. The movement of that radiopaque material is then viewed via X-ray.

Abdominal CAT scan. A CAT scan may be done if you have chronic pain to see if there are any abdominal abnormalities.

Colonic transit time. This test measures the time it takes for ingested material to move through the bowel. You take a small amount of a radioactive material, and then after five days an X-ray is taken of your bowel to see how much of the radioactive marker remains. Typically, 80 percent of the material should be gone in five days' time.

Similarities to other illnesses

ruling out other conditions

As your doctor reviews your symptoms and looks at your test results, she will begin to line up the possible disorders that match your symptoms. Unfortunately, there are many disorders that can cause gastrointestinal distress. Your doctor will need time to eliminate each possibility one by one until finally settling on the one that fits your symptoms. Only then can the correct treatment begin. The following gastrointestinal disorders, while they share symptoms with IBS, each call for their own targeted therapy.

Celiac disease is a food allergy to the protein gluten, found in grains such as wheat, oats, rye, and barley. Several symptoms of celiac disease mimic those of IBS, namely recurring abdominal bloating and pain, chronic diarrhea, gas, and fatigue. Unlike IBS, celiac disease can cause significant damage to the stomach lining as well as malnutrition. This in turn can lead to osteoporosis, because your body is not absorbing necessary nutrients. In additional to abdominal pain, celiac disease is diagnosed by pain in the joints, muscle cramps, and unexplained **anemia**, or low blood count of red cells. It may be linked to IBS, however; some studies show that celiac disease is finally diagnosed in 6 to 30 percent of patients previously and incorrectly classified as having IBS.

GERD, or gastroesophageal reflux disease, is marked by a burning sensation in your chest or throat, otherwise known as heartburn, which can sometimes also accompany IBS. Heartburn occurs when the lower esophageal sphincter, a kind of valve between your esophagus and your stomach, doesn't close properly. Ideally, food travels only one way—down the esophagus. But if that valve doesn't close properly, stomach acid and partially digested contents from your stomach can leak back, or reflux, into your esophagus. Sometimes you can even taste this "backwash" in the back of your mouth, a symptom called acid indigestion. Because heartburn is sometimes associated with IBS, it is a good idea to be evaluated for GERD. (GERD can also be caused by a hiatal hernia—when the junction between the stomach, the esophagus, and some portion of the stomach is displaced above the diaphragm.) Treatment calls for acid-inhibiting medication. If that doesn't work, then an endoscopy may be done.

Parasites are organisms that take up long-term shelter in your intestines should you ingest contaminated food or water. They can cause chronic symptoms that are similar to those of IBS, namely diarrhea, gas, and bloating. To rule out parasites, your stool needs to be tested for their presence. One common parasite called *Giardia* is known to campers and hunters who inadvertently drink contaminated water. Special antibiotics are effective against parasites.

Peptic ulcers happen when the stomach lining is injured, usually from ingesting excessive amounts of aspirin, NSAIDs (such as Ibuprofen or Motrin), caffeine, or alcohol, all of which can make it vulnerable to the corrosive action of its own natural secretion of stomach acid. Peptic ulcers can also be caused by bacteria. Regardless of the cause, the symptoms are the same (and a bit similar to those of IBS), namely stomach pain, usually after eating a meal. In some cases, doctors will also request an endoscopy (see page 11), which allows them to view the inside of the stomach lining. Sometimes biopsies of the stomach are taken during an endoscopy to determine if the ulcer is caused by bacteria, such as *H. pylori*.

Similarities continued
more disorders to rule out

Diverticulosis is an abnormal bulging out of the tiny sacs, or diverticula, that normally line the colon. This can cause abdominal pain. It is diagnosed with a colonoscopy. Treatment calls for increased fiber in the diet. **Diverticulitis** is a disease where these tiny sacs become inflamed or infected. The symptoms, which can include abdominal pain, fever, and chills, are similar to those of IBS, but much more severe. No one knows exactly what causes diverticulitis, but the theory is that high pressure on weak areas of the intestinal walls causes sacs to develop. Diverticulitis is treated with antibiotics; severe attacks may require surgery.

Ulcerative colitis affects the mucosa, or lining, of the colon and can sometimes look like IBS. Ulcerative colitis usually starts in the rectum and sigmoid colon, then extends up into the entire colon, damaging the lining. The main symptoms of ulcerative colitis are lower-abdominal pain, rectal spasms, bloody diarrhea, or pus and mucus in the stool. These bowel symptoms may be accompanied by fever, an elevated white blood cell count, nausea, vomiting, weight loss, weakness, or anorexia. Your doctor will do a colonoscopy and take a biopsy of colon tissue to confirm the diagnosis.

Crohn's disease usually involves the ileum (the lower part of the small intestine) and the colon, although it may also affect any part of the GI tract, from the mouth to the anus. Unlike ulcerative colitis, which affects only the lining of the colon, Crohn's disease can spread to nearby organs. Its symptoms, which can mimic those of IBS, can include abdominal pain and diarrhea following a meal, fever, flatulence, nausea, rectal bleeding (usually mild), frequent bowel movements, and weight loss. Diagnosis is confirmed by endoscopic tests and biopsies. Note: Both ulcerative colitis and Crohn's disease are also called inflammatory bowel disease.

Colorectal cancer, also known as colon cancer, is a slow-growing cancer that usually begins as a **polyp** (a small, noncancerous growth) on the mucous lining (mucosa) of the colon. It can include cancers of both the large intestine (colon), which is the lower part of your digestive system, and the rectum, which is the last 8 to 10 inches of your colon. Colon cancer may have no obvious symptoms in the early stages, but as it advances, some of its symptoms can mimic those of IBS. The typical symptoms include a change in bowel habits, diarrhea alternated by constipation, gas, blood in the stool, and bleeding during or after a bowel movement. Colon cancer is usually diagnosed by a colonoscopy. If you are over 50 or if you have a family history of colon cancer, you can dramatically reduce your overall risk of developing colorectal cancer by getting regular colonoscopies.

Ovarian cancer is rare (it affects 4 percent of women, most of whom are over 50 years of age), but it can be lethal in late stages. Early detection is vital but difficult because its symptoms, such as constipation, nausea, and bloating, are often attributed to other causes, such as IBS. Often the cancer has advanced before it's properly diagnosed. Symptoms in the advanced stages include bloating, indigestion, loss of appetite or fullness after eating even small amounts, nausea, unexplained weight loss, constipation, abdominal pain, and frequent urination. In some cases, CT scans, ultrasounds, and blood tests can help point toward a diagnosis, but a definitive diagnosis of ovarian cancer calls for a biopsy of ovarian tissue that reveals the presence of cancer cells.

Note: *Symptoms of IBS typically come and go over the course of hours or days. Symptoms that do not wax and wane but in fact worsen over time are usually signs of an organic disease. While uncommon, gastric cancer, cancer of the small bowel, and pancreatic cancer can all manifest a wide array of gastrointestinal symptoms. It is vital that you have these symptoms evaluated by a physician.*

Getting a diagnosis

it can take a long time

You have been given numerous diagnostic tests and they have all come back negative. That means there is no underlying physical (or **organic**) problem, such as a parasite or bowel disease, to explain your symptoms. Because IBS has no organic cause that has yet been identified, it is considered a **functional** disorder. This does not mean that IBS is not real or "all in your head." It simply means that the underlying cause for it has yet to be found. Since there is no known cause, doctors look to a defining pattern in your symptoms to guide them to a correct diagnosis. Because IBS-type symptoms can be so broad, a group of doctors met in Rome in 1999 to agree upon which key symptoms point to a diagnosis of the gastrointestinal disorder known as IBS. They determined a specific pain and symptom pattern and created the following criteria to be used in making a diagnosis of IBS (it is called the Rome II Diagnostic Criteria):

- Have abdominal pain or discomfort for 12 weeks or more (not necessarily consecutive weeks) in the previous 12 months Furthermore, this pain or discomfort is:
  - relieved by defecation
  - associated with a change in frequency of stools
  - associated with a change in appearance of stools

Other symptoms that support a diagnosis of IBS include:

- Fewer than three bowel movements a week
- More than three bowel movements a day
- Hard or lumpy stools
- Loose or watery stools
- Straining during bowel movement
- Sudden urgency to have a bowel movement

- ◆ Feeling of incomplete evacuation of stools
- ◆ Passing of mucus during bowel movement
- ◆ Abdominal bloating, swelling, or feeling of fullness

The Rome II criteria do not include fatigue and depression. But up to 94 percent of those with chronic severe IBS also experience depression and anxiety. Whether these emotional problems are the result of IBS or vice versa isn't clear. But researchers now know that they tend to occur together.

The good news is that IBS is not life threatening. In other words, the symptoms you are experiencing are not causing any harm to your intestines or bowel. Yes, your pain is real, but unlike pain from ulcerative colitis or colon cancer, it is not a harbinger of any degenerative diseases. The other good news is that IBS is treatable. Your goal is to manage your various symptoms as effectively as possible. For more on treatment see Chapter 4.

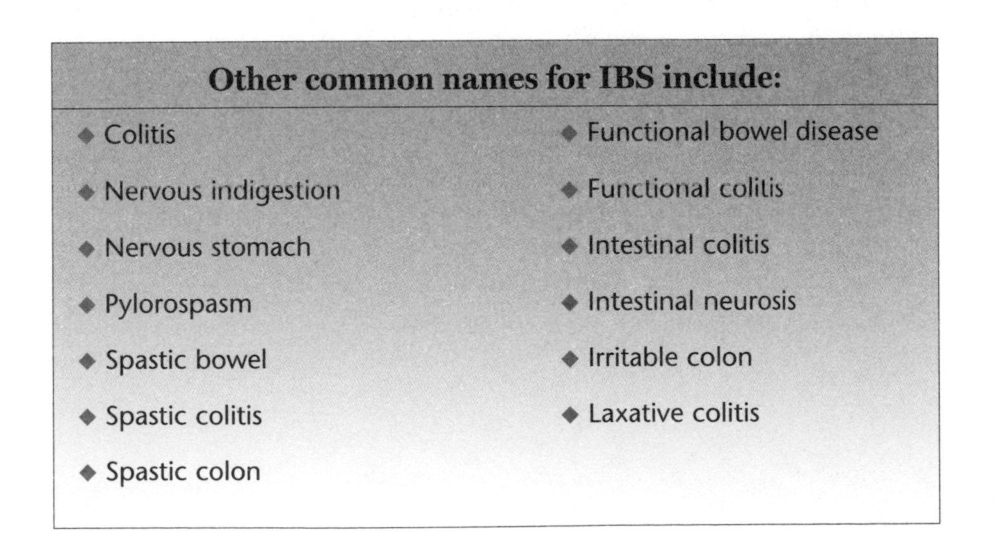

Other common names for IBS include:

- ◆ Colitis
- ◆ Nervous indigestion
- ◆ Nervous stomach
- ◆ Pylorospasm
- ◆ Spastic bowel
- ◆ Spastic colitis
- ◆ Spastic colon
- ◆ Functional bowel disease
- ◆ Functional colitis
- ◆ Intestinal colitis
- ◆ Intestinal neurosis
- ◆ Irritable colon
- ◆ Laxative colitis

Types of IBS

not all IBS is created equal

One reason IBS is so difficult to diagnose and took so long to be recognized as a viable medical disorder is that it can manifest in different ways. Some people may have constant diarrhea. Others suffer from painful constipation. Still others have pain or abdominal bloating along with bowel irregularities. Over time, doctors have identified three main forms of IBS. The form you have will help determine how you are treated, even which medications are prescribed.

Pain-predominant IBS. With this form of IBS, patients have relatively normal bowel movements and frequency, but suffer primarily from painful abdominal cramps and bloating.

Diarrhea-predominant IBS. This form of IBS is characterized by loose stools passed with urgency and with minimal straining. The diarrhea rarely occurs at night. Other common symptoms include pain and bloating, and some stool incontinence may occur.

Constipation-predominant IBS. This form of IBS is characterized by hard stools, straining during bowel movements, and incomplete evacuation. People with this form may also have some urgency and bowel frequency. The stool often contains clear or white mucus. The pain either comes in bouts or is a continuous dull ache that may improve with a bowel movement. Eating commonly triggers symptoms, which can also include bloating, flatulence, nausea, and heartburn.

Some researchers think there is another sub-type of IBS that alternates between bouts of diarrhea and constipation.

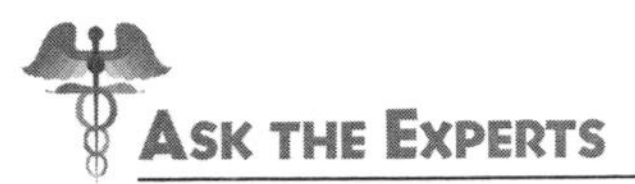

Ask the Experts

My symptoms vary. How does the doctor know which type of IBS I have?

A careful review of your symptoms will point to the type of IBS you have. While it is true that some people cycle between diarrhea and constipation, your doctor will try to find the one that occurs over 60 percent of the time. This will indicate your predominant IBS type.

Why does it matter which type of IBS I have?

Medications to treat IBS are symptom driven, e.g., antispasmodics for cramps or bulk laxatives for constipation. Some of these medications will make other IBS symptoms worse, so it is vital to diagnose the specific type of IBS you have.

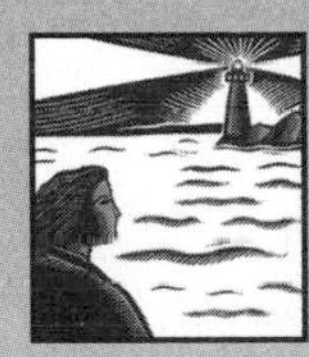

FIRST PERSON INSIGHTS

So this is IBS

When I graduated from college, I went to New York City to seek my fame and fortune. Well, it didn't quite happen that way. Instead I came down with a bad case of pelvic inflammatory disease that required massive amounts of antibiotics. My infection was gone, but a few weeks later, my stomach started acting up. I had terrible stomach cramps and constipation. At first I thought it was the stress of looking for a job, but when it continued for several more weeks, I got a little nervous. When the stomach spasms became unbearable I saw my doctor. He diagnosed IBS and prescribed some antispasmodics that I could take on an as needed basis. The pills helped get me through the really bad days. But what really helped was rest. I think my infection took a major toll on my body and I was rushing back to work too fast. I took some time off to rest and started to watch what I ate. It turned out anything really acidic like tomato sauce brought on my IBS. If nothing else, IBS has taught me to really listen to my body and take care of it. Now if I get a bout of IBS, it's because I am pushing the envelope. IBS is my signal to slow down.

—Dana L., Scarsdale, NY

Why me, why now?

what causes IBS?

As of yet, doctors don't know exactly what causes IBS. What they do know is that certain things can trigger it. In many cases, IBS starts after a gastrointestinal illness, or a course of medication (typically antibiotics), or a very stressful event. There are many things that may sensitize a person to developing IBS—some are organic, such as bacterial overgrowth, while others, such as stress, are not. Here are a few of the major culprits.

Inorganic causes

Stomach illness. Many people develop IBS after a short-term stomach infection caused by either a bacterial infection, food poisoning, or a stomach virus, such as gastroenteritis. In fact, one study found that some 10 percent of people who recovered from gastroenteritis went on to develop IBS.

Severe stress. For some people, IBS begins while they are under severe stress—coping with a family crisis, getting divorced, filing for bankruptcy, taking college exams. Researchers know there is a communication link between the brain and the intestines (or gut). Thus, severe emotional stress can cause not only depression and anxiety in the brain but IBS in the gut. (For more on this brain and gut link, see pages 72–73.) Note: Researchers have found a direct correlation between sexual abuse (emotional and/or physical) and IBS. One study showed that 50 percent of women who have severe IBS also have a history of childhood abuse. For more on this, see page 126.

Organic causes

Medication induced. Sometimes prescription medicines can bring on a case of IBS. To fight an infection, antibiotics intended to kill off the "bad" bacteria inadvertently kill off the "good" bacteria that normally live in the stomach and the bowel as well. This can greatly interfere with digestion. The antibiotic erythromycin is known to trigger IBS symptoms. Other drugs, such as diuretics, can irritate the bowel and cause IBS; so too can chemotherapy.

Bacteria overgrowth. Several intriguing studies point to an overgrowth of bacteria in the small intestine as a potential cause of IBS. These studies find that the majority of IBS study participants had excessive bacteria in the upper stomach. Treating the bacteria with the antibiotic neomycin improved symptoms of constipation, abdominal pain, diarrhea, and bowel frequency in 35 percent of the IBS participants.

Food allergies. Researchers are also looking into whether various food allergies are the culprit behind IBS. In a number of people with IBS, the inability to digest certain foods such as gluten (found in wheat), fructose (found in fruit), and lactose (found in milk products) is what is causing their IBS. In these cases, IBS is actually an inflammatory response to these allergens. In many cases, eliminating the offending food brought a halt to most, if not all, of the IBS symptoms. For more on this, see pages 66–67.

Why IBS Continues

Why doesn't your stomach return to normal after a bout of the stomach flu or once you stop taking antibiotics? As of yet, there is no known answer. What medical researchers do know is that once the digestive tract is irritated, it can take time to calm down. Since there is no disease process at work in the intestines or bowel, researchers are looking at how the brain and gut interact to affect the digestive process. Researchers think that there might be a communication breakdown between the brain and the gut that can affect how food moves through the intestines and thus trigger IBS symptoms. There is also intriguing research on how people with IBS react to pain. Studies show that those with IBS are more sensitive to pain than the norm, so that pressure in the colon that wouldn't even be noticed by someone without IBS comes across as quite painful to someone with IBS. This suggests that people with IBS may have a problem with the way pain in the colon is perceived by the brain. For more on this, see pages 72–73.

The big picture

you are not alone

Getting a diagnosis of IBS can be a bit overwhelming. On the one hand, you are glad to know that your bowel trouble has a recognized medical name, and you are thrilled to learn that it is not life threatening. But on the other hand, it is hard to hear that you have a health problem that may prove to be chronic. Yes, sure, IBS can be treated, but there will be times when it influences your quality of life. It may cushion the blow to know that you are far from alone. IBS is a far more common condition than most people know. In fact, 58 million Americans have IBS, making it more prevalent than such common disorders as asthma, diabetes, and depression. Here are some intriguing facts about IBS.

◆ IBS is a young person's illness. Half of people with IBS report having their first attack before the age of 35. The next 40 percent were between the ages of 35 and 50, while a small minority reported having their first symptoms after age 50. (Note: People who have onset of IBS symptoms after age 50 need to have a complete gastroenterological workup to rule out other conditions.)

◆ Women are far more likely than men to get IBS; 70 percent of those with IBS are women.

◆ IBS accounts for one out of every 10 doctor visits a year.

◆ IBS is the second most common reason for missing work. (Having a cold is the first.)

◆ It is estimated that one-third of those with IBS symptoms do not see a doctor, mostly because they are too embarrassed to talk about their symptoms. This is ill advised because IBS symptoms can mimic those of other serious conditions, such as inflammatory bowel disease, that call for immediate treatment.

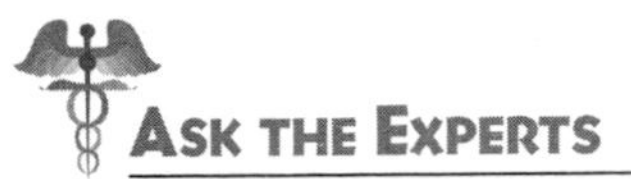

Ask the Experts

I was under a lot of stress in grad school and am pretty sure that is what brought on my IBS. Is that possible?

While severe stress (divorce, career problems, school issues) is known to trigger a number of medical conditions such as IBS, fibromyalgia, and ulcers, it is not necessarily the reason for getting them in the first place. Researchers now think that severe stress can affect areas of the body that are already predisposed toward a certain disorder or condition. For instance, those with IBS may have been born with a more sensitive gut than the norm. Severe stress may have brought that sensitivity to the forefront, but it didn't cause it.

Can my IBS worsen over time?

IBS is considered a chronic disorder that comes and goes. This waxing and waning is very stressful and may cause some people with IBS to lose their emotional resiliency. If you feel that your coping skills are diminishing, you should see your doctor and get a referral to a psychotherapist familiar with the impact of chronic illnesses on mental health. For more on this, see pages 52–53.

My IBS symptoms seem to be getting worse! Will I have to undergo those awful tests again?

There will be times when your IBS symptoms will worsen. It is the nature of the disorder—it comes and goes. To stay on top of worsening symptoms, you need to be in regular contact with your doctor (see Chapter 3 for more on health care providers). You will not have to undergo those same tests again. One full evaluation for IBS is all you need. If your symptoms continue to worsen, you need to see your doctor. Chances are you may need to take new, and most likely different, tests to rule out a potential new problem, such as cancer or an ulcer.

Keeping a health journal

listening to your body

One of the best ways to take care of yourself when you are confronted with a chronic gastrointestinal problem such as IBS is to track your health in a journal. By writing down changing symptoms you will learn how to really listen to your body and understand what it is trying to tell you. This is especially important for gastrointestinal disorders such as IBS, where you need to keep track of a number of things: what you eat, when you eat, what you were doing/thinking while you were eating, how digestion feels, and how your bowels reacted afterward.

By noting how your body responds to the entire digestive process, you can start to recognize patterns. In due time those patterns can help you and your doctor come up with a correct diagnosis. A diary will also help you identify triggers that cause flare-ups. These triggers can be anything from food to annoying people or stressful activities.

Your health journal will be very helpful to your recovery as well. How so? Treatment for IBS does not happen overnight. It sometimes takes time to determine the right combination of dietary change, stress reduction, medication, and other therapies to ease your symptoms and improve your physical and emotional functioning. By noting changes in your symptoms as you undergo them, you can plot the success of various treatments. Thus, a health journal serves as a powerful tool that can save you time and unnecessary suffering. It also does a wonderful job of reminding you that you, not your doctors, are in charge of your health.

Sample health journal

Get a three-ring binder and fill it with loose-leaf paper. Next, set aside a time every day to record how you feel. Keep it simple. Cover each major body system and identify any symptoms. Grade each symptom on a scale of 0–10, with 0 being nonexistent and 10 being a major concern. Your goal is to track the lessening or worsening of any symptoms. If you wish, make copies of the chart below and use it to find patterns to your symptoms. (For information on keeping a food diary, see pages 98–99.)

Date ______________

Type of food, drink, or medication ingested: ____________________

Last meal eaten	__________
Physical Symptoms	**0–10**
Gas/flatulence	__________
Diarrhea	__________
Constipation	__________
Incontinence	__________
Stomach/abdominal pain	__________
Stool frequency	__________
Bloated feeling	__________
Stool passage (straining, urgency, or feeling of incomplete evacuation)	__________
Mucus in stool	__________
Emotional Symptoms	
Harried/stressed	__________
Sad	__________
Angry	__________
High energy	__________
Low energy/fatigued	__________
Depressed	__________
Anxious	__________

Helpful resources

A Victim No More: Overcoming Irritable Bowel Syndrome
by Jonathan M. Berkowitz, M.D.

Understanding Irritable Bowel Syndrome
by Simon Darnley and Barbara Miller

Relief from IBS
by Elaine Fantle Shimberg

IBS: A Doctor's Plan for Chronic Digestive Troubles: The Definitive Guide to Prevention and Relief
by Gerard Guillory, M.D.

Indigestion: Living Better with Upper Intestinal Problems from Heartburn to Ulcers and Gallstones
by Henry D. Janowitz, M.D.

The Irritable Bowel Syndrome Sourcebook
by Laura O'Hare

Gut Wisdom: Understanding and Improving Your Digestive Health
by Alyce M. Sorokie

The First Year—IBS (Irritable Bowel Syndrome): An Essential Guide for the Newly Diagnosed
by Heather Van Vorous

Rome Criteria
www.romecriteria.org

Irritable Bowel Syndrome (IBS) Self Help and Support Group
www.ibsgroup.org

The Irritable Bowel Syndrome Webring
www.webring.com/hub?ring=ibs

The IBS Page
www.panix.com/~ibs

Chapter 2

How IBS Affects Your Body

Everyday digestion at work 28

Your stomach at work 30

Your bowels at work 32

Why diarrhca happens 34

Why constipation happens 36

Why gas and bloating happen 38

Helpful resources 40

Everyday digestion at work

when it's all working right

In your not-too-distant past, you probably never gave a thought to how the food you ate was digested. Not anymore. Thanks to IBS, the very act of eating can trigger your symptoms. How can that be? The answer lies in how your digestive system works.

Digestion starts in the mouth. When food or liquid enters your mouth, enzymes in your saliva immediately begin acting upon the food, breaking it down into a soft mass that can be swallowed and made ready for digestion. The more the food is broken down in the mouth, the easier it is to digest when it hits the stomach. That's why it's important that people with IBS take extra time to chew their food. For more on this, see page 97.

Swallowing is a complex coordinated act involving the tongue, muscles of the palate and the pharynx, and the esophagus—a long muscular tube leading from your throat to your stomach. At the lower end of the esophagus is a sphincter (called the LES for short), which acts as gatekeeper and allows food to travel down into the stomach. The LES must be flexible enough to also allow food to travel back up if you have eaten something that irritates the stomach (hence the ability to vomit). Sometimes this sphincter becomes too flexible and the result is a backlash of stomach acid, known as heartburn or GERD (see pages 12–13). Some people with IBS also have GERD.

Once food hits the stomach, the lining of the stomach releases hydrochloric acid and the enzyme **pepsin** to begin breaking that food down into a soft mush. (To keep from diluting pepsin and other enzymes, it is a good idea to avoid drinking fluid 30 minutes before or after eating.) Within two hours after eating, at least half of your meal should be out of your stomach. While pepsin and stomach acid work on breaking down your meal, your stomach muscles begin rhythmic contractions known as **peristalsis**. These contractions, which can sometimes be very noisy (hence the "growling" sounds of a hungry stomach) are involuntary. They are overseen by the brain/gut connection in which nerves connect the stomach wall to the brain via the spinal cord. If these nerves are in working order, they will send signals to stop eating once you are feeling full. If they misfire, they can give off wrong information, such as feelings of pain and bloating when you have eaten only a few mouthfuls of food.

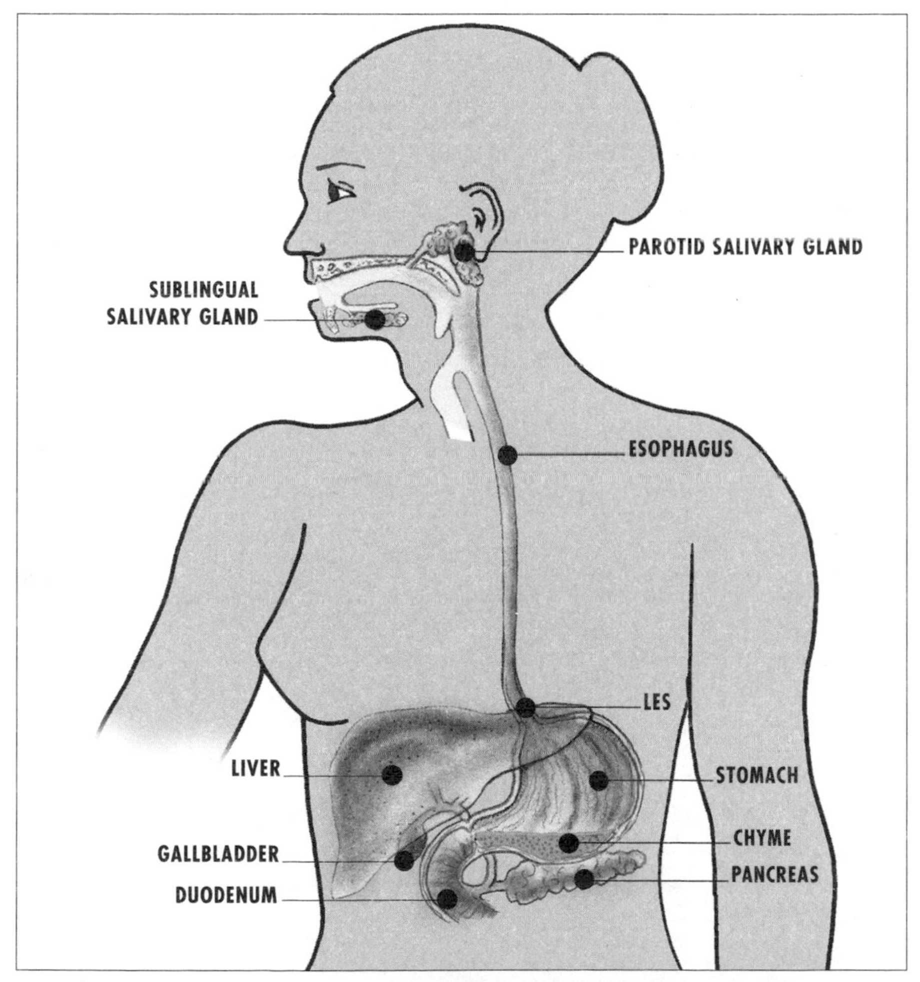

On average, the stomach can hold one quart of food per meal. To hold more food, the stomach must relax its muscles. Due to the brain-gut connection, nerves in the stomach respond directly to a stimulus from the brain and vice versa. This explains why it is hard to eat when you are upset and why it is easy to overeat when you are especially relaxed.

Your stomach at work

how food becomes fuel for your body

Once the food is in the stomach, it is mixed with digestive secretions and reduced to a semifluid substance called *chyme*. The chyme is then rhythmically driven through the pyloric sphincter into the small intestines, known as the **duodenum**, **jejunum,** and **ileum**. It is here that the chyme is digested, meaning that enzymes from the liver and pancreas are released to help convert the various nutrients in the chyme into energy: the proteins into amino acids; the carbohydrates into simple sugars; and the fats into fatty acids. Once these nutrients have been isolated, they are broken down by enzymes into molecules small enough to pass through the thin walls of the intestine into your body's bloodstream and lymph system. It is this enriched blood that feeds the cells of your body. Many things can go wrong during this nutrient-passing process. For those with diarrhea-predominant IBS,

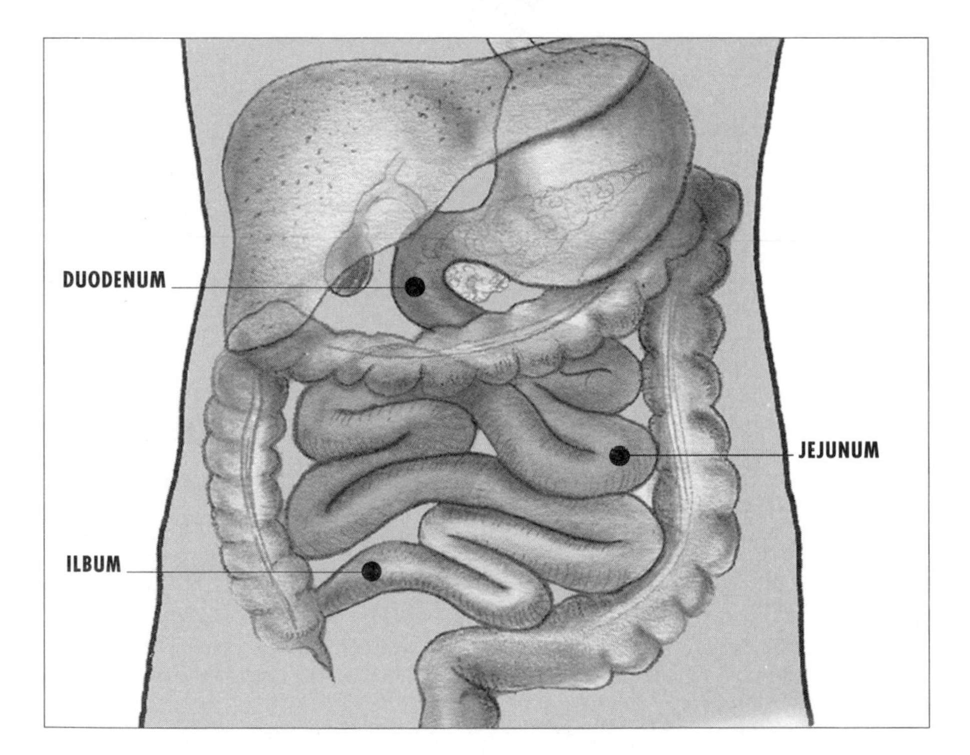

food is rushed too quickly through the intestines and there is not enough time for the nutrients to be absorbed.

Digestion requires a large surface area to do its work. The small intestines' surface area is increased by internal folds called mucosa and submucosa. These folds are topped with a velvety brush border. Inside this border are the digestive enzymes that help break down food into vital nutrients.

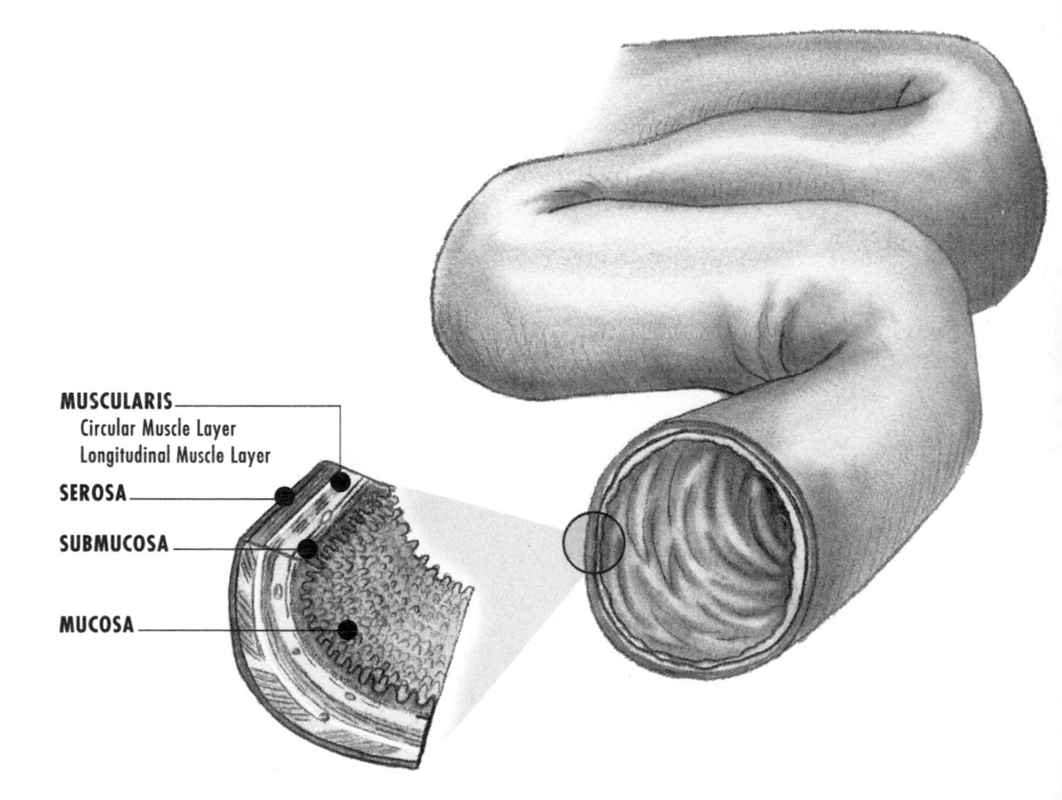

The walls of the small intestines are made up of four key layers. The outermost layer, the serosa, provides a protective coating to the lining. The next layer is the muscularis, which contains muscle fibers. On top of this muscle fiber lies the submucosa, which is composed of nerves and blood vessels. The innermost layer is the mucosa. It has millions of tiny finger-like projections called villi whose job is to absorb nutrients from the food you eat.

Your bowels at work

the last stop in digestion

Whenever matter is converted into energy, there is usually some kind of waste left behind. In your fireplace, it's ash; in your colon, it's insoluble fiber, indigestible carbohydrates, water, bile, and dead cells used up in the conversion process. In other words, fecal matter. What happens to this waste? It automatically (involuntarily) travels through the small intestine into the colon. The colon, or large intestine, is a 4-foot-long tube of muscle that is 3 inches wide. Its walls are spongy so it can soak up nearly 90 percent of the water in this leftover waste. In fact, the colon absorbs on average about 1.5 to 2 quarts of liquid each day.

The colon has additional functions, thanks to some 500 different types of bacteria that reside there. They serve a number of functions, from digesting those last bits of protein and carbohydrate to stopping any harmful bacteria from taking up residence in your bowel. One of the reasons why antibiotics can cause diarrhea is they inadvertently kill off some of these healthy bacteria. For more on this, see pages 70–71. As food residue is converted into fecal matter or stool, it undergoes slow rhythmic contractions of the colon muscle walls. This movement, or motility, of the stool is called **colonic transit time** and is a key problem to those with IBS. If it is too fast, the result is diarrhea; too slow and the result is constipation.

What triggers the release of stool? As the fecal matter accumulates in the rectum (an 8-inch-long tube at the end of the colon), the rectal wall becomes enlarged and signals the urge for a bowel movement, called the defecation reflex. The stool is ultimately released by the sphincter in the anus. Unlike the esophagus sphincter, there is a portion of the anus function that is under voluntary control.

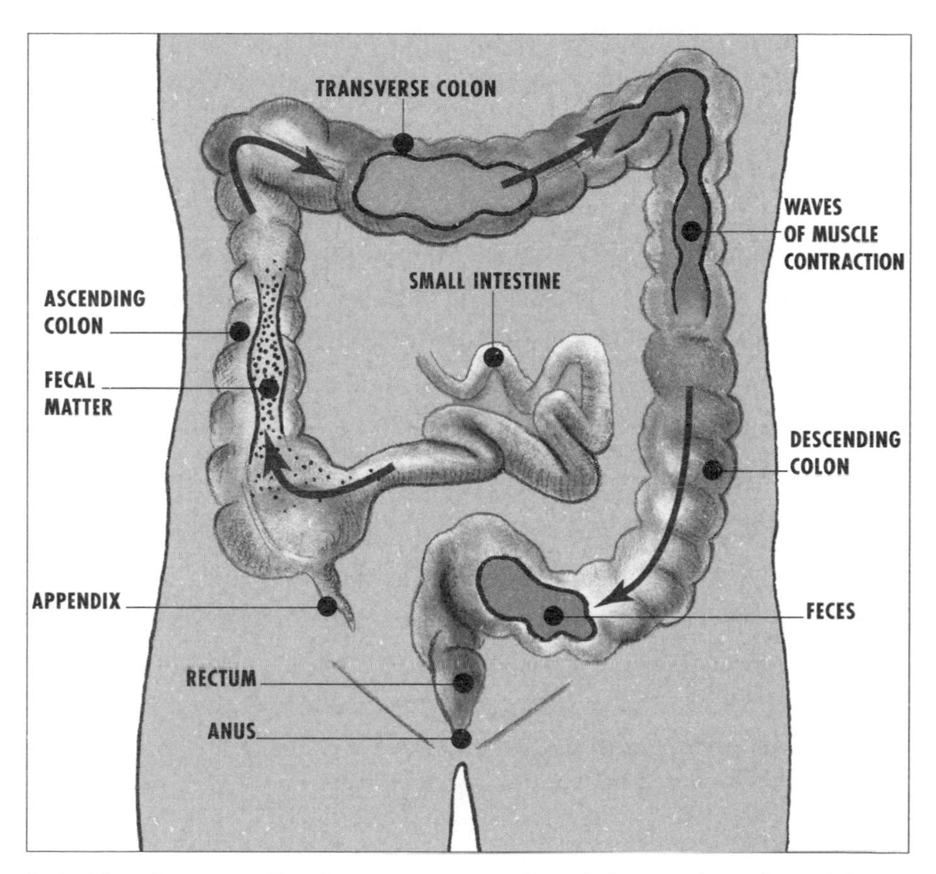

Peristaltic actions moves digestive watery waste up through the ascending colon and then over to the transverse colon, where more and more of its water is absorbed by the colon. Then the waste officially turns into stool matter and moves down the descending colon and into the rectum.

A question many people with IBS want to ask their doctors but are too embarrassed to is: What does a normal bowel movement look like? A normal bowel movement, which can range in size, should be easy and effortless to pass. The lighter the color of the stools, the better. Darker colored and heavier stools are the result of a high protein diet. A simple wipe of toilet paper should suffice; if more paper is needed, then you may have greasy stools, which are a sign that fats are not being digested. There should not be a lot of odor when the bowel movement is finished, and there should be a sense that the bowel movement is complete.

Why diarrhea happens

when the system overreacts

Your digestive tract is designed to cope with various mishaps, such as spoiled food or the occasional stomach virus or bacterial infection. In such cases, it reacts with a protective mechanism that rejects the contents of the stomach by either vomiting it out or ejecting it rapidly via diarrhea. In order to rid itself of any remnants of the offender, the stomach repeats this uncomfortable process until the culprit is gone and the crisis has passed—typically in a few days. Your digestive tract then goes back to its normal state of affairs. But sometimes it doesn't work that way. In some 20 percent of those with persistent IBS symptoms, an acute bacterial infection was the trigger.

In IBS, chronic diarrhea is essentially a problem of too rapid a colonic transit time. In other words, the watery waste matter is pushed by the bowel muscles too quickly through the bowel and there is not enough time to absorb the liquid from it. The result is cramps and diarrhea. Why does this continue to happen? Researchers are not quite sure. One theory puts the blame on a faulty brain/gut connection. The brain and gut share a special messenger cell called serotonin. In the brain, the lack of it causes depression; in the stomach—or so the theory goes—the lack of it may interfere with colonic transit time. Still another theory blames stress. Since stress is known to deplete serotonin in the brain, surely it must affect the stomach's serotonin, too. (Occasionally food intolerances, such as lactose intolerance, result in incomplete digestion and too quick a transit time through the gut.) Theories abound. The good news is that there *is* treatment for IBS with predominant diarrhea; see page 120.

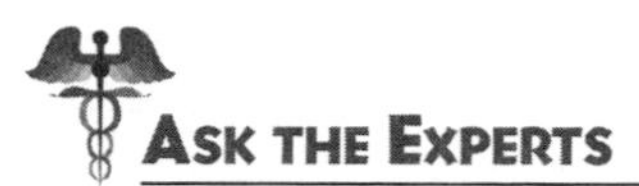

Ask the Experts

I have predominant diarrhea IBS and my doctor has urged me to try the BRAT diet. Why do these foods help against diarrhea?

The "BRAT" diet is the abbreviation for a short-term diet that consists of bananas, rice, apples, and toast. It is commonly suggested to people who are undergoing an acute (short-term) bout of diarrhea. It works because these four foods are lactose-free and provide fiber and some potassium. The BRAT diet is not good for the long-term management of IBS.

How do over-the-counter remedies work against short-term diarrhea?

Some over-the-counter medicines (such as Pepto-Bismol) contain bismuth, a substance that helps stomach secretions. Others (such as Imodium and Kaopectate) contain loperamide, which decreases the movement in the digestive tract and slows the colonic transit time.

My doctor suggested I take extra fiber to help stop my diarrhea. I thought fiber was only for constipation.

Fiber is extremely effective for both constipation and diarrhea. Because fiber helps absorb water in the stool, it adds bulk to the stool and thus slows down colonic transit time. For this reason, most doctors consider it the most important therapy for diarrhea. For more on fiber, see pages 100–101.

My pharmacist told me about probiotics to help with my diarrhea. What are probiotics?

Diarrhea tends to wipe out the healthy bacteria in the colon. How to replace that good bacteria? Enter probiotics. These are live bacterial cultures you can take, either by eating yogurt or in pill form, that will help replenish your eradicated bacteria. The theory is that probiotics will help balance out your digestive system. For more on probiotics, see pages 70–71.

Why constipation happens

when the system slows down

This may surprise you, but constipation is a very common complaint that affects 20 percent of the population every day. The problem with constipation is that it can be somewhat subjective. Some perfectly healthy people move their bowels once a day; some do it a few times a week. It's changes in your normal bowel habits that signal constipation-predominant IBS. Try to think back to the times before your IBS struck. What was your general pattern? That is what would be considered your personal "normal."

In medical terms, constipation is defined as defecating less than three times a week and passing hard stools and/or straining from one to three out of four times you move your bowels, or a decrease in frequency in your normal pattern. Why does it happen? There a number of reasons. The most common ones are not enough liquids or fiber in your diet—liquid makes stools easier to pass while fiber makes them softer. Another reason could be certain medications that have constipation as a side effect. For example, most narcotic painkillers slow down the muscles in the central nervous system, and that includes the stomach and bowel muscles. Another reason for constipation is lack of exercise. Exercise gets all your muscles moving, including your stomach and pelvic muscles, which are involved in digestion and defecation.

In constipation-predominant IBS, the reason for constipation is usually slow colonic transit time. Meaning, fecal matter is moving too slowly through the colon. When this happens, nearly all the fecal matter's water is absorbed by the colon so that what is left is hard and pelletlike. Again, there is treatment for both types of IBS—chronic constipation (see page 120) and constipation with diarrhea (see page 120).

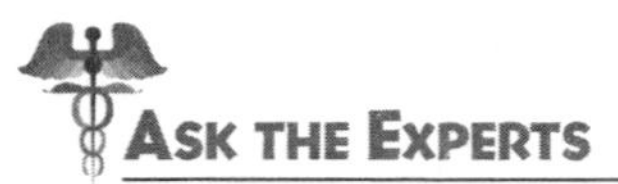

I have been using laxatives for years and now my doctor wants to get me off of them. How will I manage?

Misuse of over-the-counter laxatives is pretty common. The reason your doctor wants you to stop them is that she needs to know how your bowels work on their own. Another reason is that part of your IBS treatment calls for training your bowels to work more effectively. Yes, your bowels can be trained. For example, people who are constipated often put off going to the bathroom; this teaches your bowels to stop registering the urge to go.

Why does fiber help with constipation?

Fiber helps fecal matter hold on to water as it passes through the colon, so it makes passing the stool easier and faster. And fiber also adds bulk to feces, so that more is evacuated. There are two types of fiber supplements: insoluble fiber, such as bran, and soluble fiber, such as psyllium, the pectins in fruit. Some soluble fiber is digested by colon bacteria, which can create gas and bloating. Both types will help speed up colon transit time. (Note: Some foods contain both types of fiber.)

Sources of Insoluble Fiber	Sources of Soluble Fiber
Wheat bran	Oat bran
Corn bran	Whole oats
Whole grains	Rice bran
Dried beans and peas	Dried beans
Popcorn	Chickpeas, black-eyed peas, and lentils
Seeds and nuts	All fruits
Most fruits	All vegetables
Most vegetables, especially carrots, white potatoes, broccoli, leeks, and parsnips	

Why gas and bloating happen

what causes these painful sensations

There are two types of gastrointestinal gas. Gas that comes from the mouth in the form of a belch or burp is due to swallowed air that forces itself back out. Eating while talking often results in burps; so can chewing gum and smoking. The other type of gas is the kind that comes out of the rectum. It is essentially the byproduct of the digestive processes going on in the colon. The bacteria in the colon can be very active. They digest any left-over proteins and carbohydrates in the food residue sent to the colon. The nutrients they glean from this process are used to keep the colon tissue healthy. In this final stage of the digestive process, gas, typically carbon dioxide, hydrogen, and methane gas, is emitted. This is a normal and natural byproduct of digestion. Certain foods, such as beans, are known to create excess gas. This is because the carbohydrates in beans cannot be broken down in the intestines; only the colon can handle them.

Bloating is what happens when the digestive gases in the colon are not readily released. But like IBS, bloating turns out to be something of a pain-perception problem. People who complain of bloat are not necessarily experiencing more gas than normal; rather, their stomachs are overly sensitive to gas pain, causing the intestines to spasm and move the chyme in the wrong direction. All this activity results in a feeling of bloat. The good news is that while everyday bloating is uncomfortable, it is not necessarily a sign of a health problem. (Severe bloating, however, needs to be evaluated by a doctor to rule out such serious health problems as Crohn's disease or a bowel obstruction.)

Coping with Bloating and Gas

Gas is a natural byproduct of digestion. A little bit of gas here and there is perfectly normal, especially if you have eaten something that creates a lot of gas in the colon, such as beans or vegetables from the cabbage family. Too much gas is uncomfortable, not to mention embarrassing. Here are some tips to stop the problem before it starts:

◆ Eat slowly and chew with your mouth closed so you do not swallow a lot of air as you eat. Try not to talk excitedly during a meal; this usually results in swallowed air—which ultimately becomes gas.

◆ Stand up and stretch or go for a walk after eating. This helps move the food through the digestive system and can more easily move the gas along and out.

◆ Eliminate all carbonated beverages.

◆ Rid your diet of all beans, cabbage, and corn. They're top gas producers.

◆ Stay away from sorbitol. This artificial sweetener, found in soft drinks, gum, etc., is hard to digest and can result in gas. Also, avoid lactulose, a synthetic sugar used in prescription medicine for constipation.

◆ Cut out caffeine, a known colon irritant.

Helpful resources

Understanding Irritable Bowel Syndrome
by Simon Darnley and Barbara Millar

The Sensitive Gut
by Michael Lasalandra, Harvard Medical School; and Lawrence Friedman

Irritable Bowel Syndrome and the MindBodySpirit Connection: 7 Steps for Living a Healthy Life with a Functional Bowel Disorder, Crohn's Disease, or Colitis
by William B. Salt II, M.D., and Neil F. Neimark, M.D.

Gut Wisdom: Understanding and Improving Your Digestive Health
by Alyce M. Sorokie

The Good Gut Guide: Help for IBS, Ulcerative Colitis, Crohn's Disease, Diverticulitis, Food Allergies, Other Gut Problems
by Stephanie Zinser

The IBS Self Help Group
www.ibsgroup.org

UNC Center for Functional GI & Motility Disorders
www.med.unc.edu/wrkunits/2depts/medicine/fgidc/welcome.htm

National Institute of Diabetes & Digestive & Kidney Diseases
www.niddk.nih.gov/

IBS Resource Center at HealingWell.com
www.healingwell.com/ibs

Irritable Bowel Information & Support Association of Australia
www.ibis-australia.org

CHAPTER 3

Your Support Team

Creating a health team 42

Your primary care doctor 44

Your gastroenterologist 46

Your pharmacist 48

Your dietitian 50

Working with a therapist 52

Your advocate 54

Using your health journal 56

How to be a smart patient 58

Joining a support group 60

Helpful resources 62

Creating a health team

take charge of your health

While it's understandable that you may not feel up to taking an active, ongoing role in making decisions about your irritable bowel syndrome, you really do need to try to take center stage. Even if you were raised in an era in which patients never questioned a doctor's word, you need to regard the doctors who treat you more as consultants than cure-all healers who have all the answers. The reason for this is simple: The more you are involved in your care and treatment, the more likely you are to see positive results.

When it comes to IBS there is much that is not known and you need to surround yourself with health professionals who are willing to explore new ideas and theories with you. Your team can range from a gastroenterologist (see page 46) to a dietitian (see page 50) to a mental health therapist (see page 52). Bear in mind that you're seeking professionals who share your values and philosophies about IBS. You don't want someone who thinks your pain is "all in your head." Instead, you need to feel comfortable with the members of your team and confident in their ability to treat you. Conversely, they need to be willing to listen to you and consider your input and suggestions.

Creating a Partnership

Good relationships with health professionals require effort on both sides. Just as you have rights and responsibilities as a patient, your doctor has certain rights and responsibilities. As with any relationship, the doctor-patient one rests on respect and trust. It's a true partnership. In that partnership, you are entitled to

- Be fully informed about your diagnosis, prognosis, and treatment
- Have a say in decisions affecting your health
- Have all your questions and concerns dealt with
- Have your medical records released only with your consent
- Have reasonable access to your doctor
- Be told about the costs and risks of treatment
- Change doctors, request a referral, or get a second opinion
- Be seen within a reasonable amount of time
- Be told how a test or procedure works, how much it costs, and what the alternatives and risks are before consenting to treatment

In return, your doctor has certain rights as well. These include the right to

- Be treated with courtesy
- Be allowed enough time to make a diagnosis
- Have her advice followed carefully
- Be notified in a timely manner if you must cancel or change an appointment

Your primary care doctor

know what you want from your family doctor

Your primary care doctor, who may be a family practitioner or general internist, is probably the one who diagnosed your IBS in the first place. She picked up on your symptoms, suggested possible diagnoses, and worked with you to finally put a name to the painful and uncomfortable symptoms you'd been having for months or even years.

She will serve as a kind of captain of your medical team, directing your care and maintaining a "big picture" approach to your condition and treatment. It is important that all other members of your team communicate regularly with her. One way to ensure that this occurs is to give all the other members of your team permission to share your medical information with her, providing them with her full name, phone number, e-mail, and mailing address, as well as your signature of consent.

You will also need to continue seeing your primary care doctor for non-IBS-related issues, like infections and other illnesses.

However, if none of the IBS treatments your primary care doctor prescribes seem to work, you have other gastrointestinal problems in addition to IBS, or you just want a second opinion or someone else to take a look at your case, you may want to consider seeing an IBS specialist called a gastroenterologist.

Don't worry about offending your primary care doctor. She knows that she is a generalist and that sometimes specialists are necessary. In fact, she may be the one to suggest you see a specialist!

Choosing a Primary Care Physician

Frustrated by your primary care doctor's inability to find a reason for your painful bowel movements, diarrhea, and gas, you decide to find another doctor. Or you've just moved into a new area and need to find a new physician. This is a big decision because anyone with a chronic health condition, like you, develops a very close relationship with his or her doctor.

To find a new physician, start by talking to people you know. Ask your friends and family about their own primary care physicians—why they like the doctor, what the doctor is like to work with. Also check with anyone you know who has IBS. If you don't know anyone, look in the newspaper or call your local hospital for information on IBS support groups. Group members may have experience with good physicians for your condition. Additionally, most hospital systems have physician referral lines. They may be able to put you in touch with someone who specializes in digestive problems yet still maintains a general practice.

Once you find a doctor, schedule an appointment. (Doctors do not do interviews.) See how you like that new doctor before transferring over your medical records. Expect to pay for this first visit.

Remember that under the Health Insurance Portability and Accountability Act that took effect in April 2003 you have the right to a copy of your medical records. Before you switch doctors, get a copy and correct any errors and then keep a copy in your health journal. Make several duplicates, to give to your new primary care physician and other doctors you may see. This will save a great deal of time.

Your gastroenterologist

your second line of defense

Some people with IBS don't get a diagnosis until they see a **gastroenterologist**, a doctor who specializes in diseases and disorders of the digestive system. A gastroenterologist is an internist who has completed an additional three years of fellowship training in the digestive system, spending the third year gaining a subspecialty in one of several areas: advanced endoscopy, liver transplant, motility (or the movement of substances through the intestines), inflammatory bowel disease, the esophagus, or nutrition and metabolism. Ideally you should find a doctor with a subspecialty in motility, since he will likely see the most cases of IBS. Any gastroenterologist, however, is qualified to treat you.

To find a gastroenterologist, first start with your family doctor. Most gastroenterologists receive patient referrals from community family doctors who are used to working closely with specialists. Also talk to friends and family about any gastroenterologists they may have seen in the past.

During your first appointment, spend a few minutes talking about his practice philosophy. Ask how he treats other IBS patients in his practice, and what kind of success he's had with the treatment plans he follows. Listen carefully not only to what the doctor says, but to what you feel in your gut. Remember the brain in your gut? It comes in handy now as you decide whether this is a person you feel comfortable with and can work closely with.

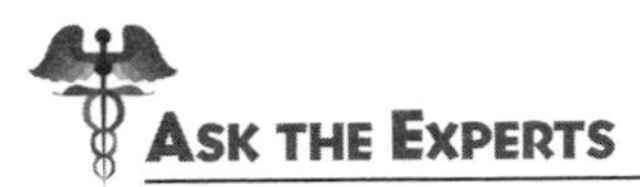

My primary care physician has already run a lot of tests on me. Will the specialist repeat them all?

It depends on what tests were run and when they were done. If it's been a while, a gastroenterologist may want to repeat them to check the results. Generally, however, the new doctor should be able to view the results of all tests in your medical chart without having to repeat them.

Questions to Ask Specialists

Although it's highly unlikely that you will talk to the doctor before your first appointment, asking the doctor's nurse or even receptionist some pertinent questions can help you get a better feel for how the doctor operates and how the office is run. These include:

- How long has the doctor been specializing in IBS?
- What percentage of the doctor's practice is composed of IBS patients?
- Does the doctor use an integrated approach, combining both traditional medical therapies and complementary medicine?
- How much does the doctor charge for a consultation?
- What insurances does the doctor accept?
- What type of information should I bring to the first appointment? How long does the first evaluation take?
- What is the typical waiting time in your office?
- At which hospitals does the doctor practice?

Your pharmacist

the "safety net" in managing your illness

Prescription medication as well as over-the-counter medicine is often used to manage IBS. That's why it's a good idea to develop a relationship with your pharmacist. Your pharmacist can act as a "safety net" in managing your prescriptions, not only for your IBS medicine but for any possible interactions with other medications as well.

The best strategy is to fill all your prescriptions at the same place so you get to know the pharmacist there and he or she gets to know you and your record. Also, using one pharmacist and pharmacy makes it easier to keep your medication records up to date. Some pharmacies can even provide a printout of the medications you're taking, along with their dosages and potential interactions—valuable information to have with you at all times.

Pharmacists are also terrific resources for information about over-the-counter medications and alternative therapies and supplements. In fact, they usually know more about possible interactions between supplements and prescription medications than doctors do.

If you use impersonal drug chains for your medication needs or order most of your drugs online or via mail, then make sure you schedule an annual drug check with your primary care doctor. During this appointment, you bring in all the medications you're taking and your doctor reviews them to make sure you still need each one in the prescribed dose.

Always double-check with your pharmacist about when and how to take your medications, and make sure these instructions match the instructions on the bottle.

Buying Medications Online

While some Web sites offer great prices on prescription drugs, not all such sites are legitimate. The National Association of Boards of Pharmacy (NABP) offers the following advice about purchasing prescription drugs online:

◆ It is risky to buy medication from illegal Web sites. You may receive a contaminated or counterfeit product, the wrong product, an incorrect dose, or no product at all.

◆ Purchasing drugs that aren't normally available in the U.S. can be a very dangerous experiment with your own health. It's also illegal. If you get ripped off, no U.S. agency can do anything to help you resolve the issue.

◆ Getting a prescription drug by filling out a questionnaire without seeing a health care professional puts you at serious risk. You may end up with a drug that is unsafe for you or one that may not be the best for you.

◆ Check the legitimacy of a drug-dispensing Web site on the VIPPS (Verified Internet Pharmacy Practice Sites) page at the National Association of Boards of Pharmacy Web site at **www.nabp.net** or by calling the NABP at 847-698-6227.

◆ Do business only with Web sites that allow you direct access to a registered pharmacist to answer your questions. When you receive the medication, ask the site's pharmacist all the same questions you would ask your local drugstore pharmacist.

◆ If you use a drug-dispensing Web site, it's up to you to monitor your medications for any potential adverse interactions. Tell your regular pharmacist about any drugs you've purchased online when filling new prescriptions in person.

Your dietitian

help with eating right

Because IBS is a condition of the digestive system, it is intimately influenced by what, when, and how you eat (see Chapter 6). For this reason, and many others, it is a good idea to add a registered dietitian or nutritionist to your treatment team.

The American Dietetic Association defines a **registered dietitian** (RD) as a highly trained food and nutrition expert who has met minimum academic and professional requirements. These include a bachelor's degree with courses in food and nutrition sciences, food service systems management, business, economics, computer science, sociology, biochemistry, physiology, microbiology, and chemistry and an accredited, supervised, six- to 12-month internship at a health-care facility, community agency or food service corporation. Additionally, an RD must pass a national examination administered by the Commission on Dietetic Registration and continue her professional education.

Most registered dietitians work at hospitals and medical centers, in private practices, or in other health care facilities. Many work in community and public health settings, academia, and research.

A dietitian will ask about your eating habits, IBS, and nutritional lifestyle. For instance, if you tend to eat lunch out or travel a great deal, that's important information and will play a role in the dietary plan the RD designs for you. She will then help you set reasonable goals for your eating habit and will develop eating plans for you, both for dining at home and on the road and in restaurants. She can recommend foods that won't exacerbate your IBS and that will help you avoid any food-related intolerances or allergies, even while maintaining a healthy nutritional profile. Don't forget to bring your health journal with you to your appointment.

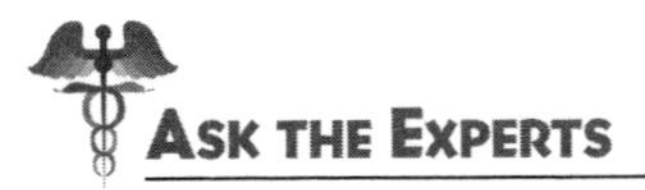

Ask the Experts

What is a registered dietetic technician?

Dietetic technicians, registered (DTRs), often work in partnership with registered dietitians to screen, evaluate, and educate patients, manage and prevent diseases such as diabetes and obesity, and monitor the progress of a patient or client. They must complete at least a two-year associate's degree in an approved dietetics technology program from an accredited U.S. college or university, have supervised practice experience in community programs, health care and food service facilities, pass a nationwide examination, and continue taking education courses throughout their careers.

Working with a therapist

help with the stress of life and IBS

If you feel that the simple fact of living with irritable bowel syndrome puts more stress on you than you can easily handle, you are not alone. And chances are you may also feel that issues in your current or past life are making your IBS symptoms worse. Talking to a professional therapist is one of the best things you can do.

Finding the right therapist can take some time. Talk to your primary care physician and to friends and family about therapists they've seen. Most therapists will agree to an initial visit—sometimes without charge—to see if the two of you can work together. It's extremely important that you feel you can trust this person; you're going to be talking about some very intimate and possibly painful issues with her. If you don't feel comfortable and can't open up, you're just wasting your time and money.

Try to find a therapist experienced in working with people who have chronic diseases. Often, a local support group or your hospital can recommend such a person.

Sorting Through the Therapy Alphabet Soup

Anyone can hang out a shingle and call herself a therapist. You should look for someone licensed as a therapist by your state, with, at the very least, an advanced degree. Here's what you need to know about what the various degrees really mean.

M.A./M.S. (Master of Art/Science). This person has usually completed one to three years of postgraduate study, including an internship.

L.P.C. (Licensed Professional Counselor). In some states, therapists who are licensed will have these initials after their name.

Ph.D. (Doctor of Philosophy). This therapist has completed five or more years of postgraduate study, including writing a dissertation or original research. Obviously, you want someone whose Ph.D. is in a clinical area, such as psychology or counseling. The Ph.D. often focuses more on research and teaching than on clinical work, however.

Psy.D. (Doctor of Psychology). This is a professional psychology degree requiring about five or more years of full-time postgraduate study. In contrast to Ph.D.'s, Psy.D.'s focus on developing clinical skills rather than research or teaching.

Ed.D. (Doctor of Education). Doctoral level degree in school psychology with specific training focused on working with teachers, parents, and students on learning, behavioral, or emotional problems in the school setting.

M.F.C. (Marriage and Family Counselor) or M.F.C.C. (Marriage, Family, and Child Counselor). This therapist usually has a Master's degree and is licensed by the state. Specifically trained in dealing with family, marital, and parent-child conflicts and problems.

L.C.S.W., C.S.W., M.S.W. (social workers). You're most likely to see this kind of therapist. Their focus is on helping healthy individuals cope with current, time-limited problems. An L.C.S.W. is a licensed clinical social worker, while a C.S.W. or M.S.W. has not necessarily received training in therapeutic techniques. So always ask about their specific training and area of expertise.

M.D. (Doctor of Medicine). These professionals have attended medical school and completed a residency in psychiatry. Unlike other therapists, they can write prescriptions for medication. You may find that you see a psychologist or other nonmedical therapist for actual talk therapy and an M.D. only if you need medication to treat anxiety, depression, or some other mental illness.

Your advocate

when you need emotional support

As you build your health care team, don't forget one of the most important elements: your personal advocate, or coach. This could be a family member or a friend—someone who can help you navigate the medical maze. Your advocate should be open minded, a good listener, and above all, someone who respects your confidence.

Your advocate should serve as a sounding board for the emotional ups and downs you will face as you learn to live with a chronic illness. He or she should also be willing to help you with practical matters, such as going to doctor's appointments with you or running errands for you when you're having an IBS flare-up.

Other things your advocate can do:

- Stay informed about your illness, symptoms, and medications by conducting online searches
- Speak up for you at doctor visits when you feel the doctor doesn't understand what you're trying to say
- Take notes on what the doctor or other health professional tells you after an examination, so you can focus on just listening
- Help you track your medications and encourage you to continue the healthy habits you're struggling to maintain
- Help you cope with the paperwork and medical bills that accompany any chronic medical condition
- Help you keep your sense of humor

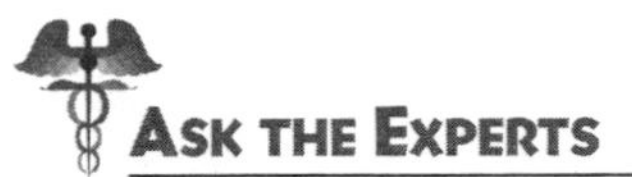

Ask the Experts

Ever since my diagnosis of IBS, my best friend has become distant. It's almost like she doesn't want to be around me. Why is she acting like this?

Your friend's distance may be due to the fact that she doesn't know what to say or how to help you. Because she feels unable to help, she backs away. If that is the case, then there are things you can do. Invite her for lunch or tea so you can talk about how much you enjoy her company. Take some time and explain what IBS is about and how it affects your life. Make it clear that although you may have bad days, you still need her and value her friendship as much as—if not more than—ever, and that your IBS should not adversely color your friendship.

As my IBS has gotten worse, I've found it more difficult to get out of the house and join my friends in the activities we used to share. I just don't feel up to hitting the bars or going dancing these days. Yet I miss my friends. What can I do?

One of the hardest parts of having IBS is always having to be near a bathroom because you just don't know when you will have to go. One very simple solution is to plan events at your own home. How about hosting a potluck dinner in your own house or apartment? You can ask everyone to bring a dish, rent a few movies, and have a relaxing evening together. (Of course, you'll need to make sure there will be food you can eat that doesn't aggravate your IBS.) Another option is to plan some less strenuous activities, like taking in a movie or a play. Or see if you can get one of your friends to be your exercise buddy, since regular exercise is an important component of your IBS treatment plan (for more on exercise, see pages 114–115). A 20-minute walk with a friend can give you not only valuable exercise but much-needed social support.

Using your health journal

good information at your fingertips

Hopefully, you've been keeping your health journal (described on pages 24–25) since you started reading this book. By now, it might be quite a few pages long, covering several weeks. Well, as any CEO worth his or her weight in stock options knows, information is valuable only when you can put it to work for you. Chances are you've got valuable information in there that can help you and your team better manage your IBS.

So how do you get the information out in a usable form? You look for patterns. You can do this visually, just sitting down and going through your journal, or you can input the information into some kind of computer database. Assuming that the former is easier, here's what to look for.

Changes in sleep patterns. Are you sleeping more or less? Is your sleep restful or fitful?

Changes in pain. Is your pain worsening or lessening? Are there any precipitating factors that make the pain worse or better? Is it worse or better at various times of the day? How are you handling it? Is it changing your daily activities? In what way?

Changes in diet and digestion. Are you craving certain foods? Finding that certain foods exacerbate your IBS symptoms? Having problems digesting certain foods? Are you eating more or less? Losing weight or gaining? Eating at certain times of the day?

Changes in bathroom habits. Are you having more or fewer bowel movements? Are they more or less painful? What about urinary problems?

Life events. What kinds of life events (new job, divorce, marriage, pregnancy) have occurred over the past couple of months? Do they correlate with any changes in your symptoms?

Emotional or mood patterns. Can you pick up any patterns of feelings? For instance, if you're feeling sad every afternoon, you may have a blood-sugar problem separate from your IBS. If you have a hard time getting out of bed in the morning because you're depressed, that may signify an unhappiness with your life that a therapist can help you work through.

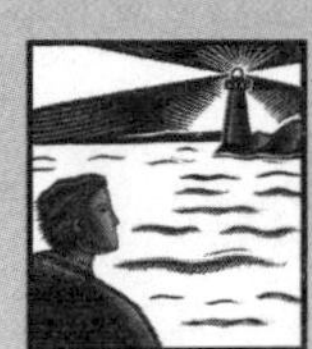

FIRST PERSON INSIGHTS

Listening to yourself

For years I felt as if my Irritable Bowel Syndrome controlled me, instead of the other way around. I never knew if my chronic digestive problems would prevent me from attending events or even going to work in the morning. Then I started keeping a health journal. I wrote down everything I ate, what I did each day, how I felt both emotionally and physically, and tracked all my symptoms. I also added a column for any remedies I tried, from medication to exercise to supplements, to see if they made a difference. Three months after I started keeping the journal, I sat down and carefully went through it. What I found amazed me. I never realized how much coffee I drank every day, but I found that on the days I had more than one cup, my symptoms were worse. I also found that if I ate fast food, my symptoms got worse, just as they did any time I had an argument with my teenage son. Recognizing these patterns has made all the difference in the world. Today, I know what to eat and how to protect myself from stressful situations that are sure to result in an IBS flare-up. Today, I control my IBS; it doesn't control me!

—Sarah M., Queens Village, NY

How to be a smart patient

making the most of your appointment

You expect a lot of the medical professionals on your treatment team. But they, in turn, expect a lot of you. If you don't take responsibility for your care seriously, you're just going to waste their time and yours.

Thus, it's important to prepare for your visit just as you'd prepare for a business meeting or conference. It's not hard to do, especially if you've been keeping your health journal as described on pages 24–25.

Leaf through your journal looking for trends and patterns as described on pages 56–57. Be sure your journal contains a record of your most recent IBS-related symptoms and full details about your day: what you ate, what you did, when the pain started, what kinds of events you were coping with, if you were under any kind of unusual stress, what you did for relief. Think of the professionals on your treatment team as your partners: The more they know about you and your condition, the better they'll be able to help you.

Have these ready on the day of your first appointment with any new health professional:

◆ Copies of medical records from prior evaluations. You can also send these to your new doctor before your appointment so he or she has a chance to review them.

◆ A list of medications you're currently taking and those you've taken in the past, along with a description of how they worked for you and any side effects you experienced.

◆ A list of questions you have about your irritable bowel syndrome. (Focus on your IBS. Save other health-related questions for another visit.)

◆ A description of your current health problem. Try to keep it short and to the point and as specific as possible. For example, "I've had abdominal pain in my lower left belly lasting two to six hours, mostly after eating. The pain is so intense that I can't walk." This is much more helpful than, "My stomach hurts."

Insurance Help

Insurance can be complicated and confusing, especially for people who need long-term treatment. It's not always clear what health services your insurance company covers for irritable bowel syndrome and other chronic conditions and for how long. For instance, if your doctor prescribes an antidepressant, will your insurance company require a diagnosis of depression before approving refills? Here are some tips to help you cope with insurance hassles:

- Call ahead to your insurance company to determine what is and isn't covered. Don't assume that insurance won't cover a particular service, such as nutritional counseling or referral before you ask. If you have severe IBS that is affecting the quality of your life, see if you can get a preauthorized health service, such as sessions with a psychologist who can help with coping strategies.

- Work with your doctor to get letters of necessity to encourage your insurance company to cover a service it initially rejected.

- Complete claim forms fully. Don't provide an excuse for having a claim form rejected.

- If a claim is initially rejected, appeal it.

- If your health insurance is provided through your employer (and you don't mind sharing some of your health information), talk to your human resources department if you're being denied care. Often, the company itself is the one paying for the services and has the flexibility to approve the care.

Joining a support group

sharing your experience with others

One of the hardest things about having a chronic illness is the feeling that you're the only one experiencing it—particularly a disorder like IBS, which can be embarrassing both to have and to talk about. The loneliness that comes from such a condition can be as difficult to you emotionally as the condition itself. But thanks to the Internet, others with your condition are just a phone call or a few keystrokes away. Finding such support is vital to your recovery: Not only will you be provided with information and resources on your condition, but you'll also discover a safe environment where you can share your experiences and get valuable support and advice.

A support group can help you deal with all the complications IBS can cause in your daily life and the anxieties it can bring on, including changing roles for family members and the feeling that you've lost control of your life. Other common issues discussed in support groups include dealing with a new diagnosis, medications, avoiding IBS triggers, and general burnout.

You'll also learn valuable everyday tips about coping with your condition. For instance, a support group is a great place to get advice on IBS-friendly dishes at chain restaurants.

Most support groups, even those online, have a facilitator who organizes the group and runs the meetings. Sometimes this is a physician, therapist, or social worker; sometimes it's someone just like you living with IBS. The facilitator not only ensures that your concerns are addressed but maintains control of the group or message board if the topic strays too far from IBS.

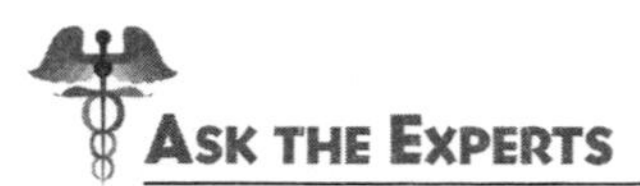

Ask the Experts

Where can I find an IBS support group in my town?

Check with your doctor. Or better yet, call your local or regional hospital (ask for its community or public relations office). It's quite likely, particularly if you live in a large urban area, that there are several IBS groups under way.

What about online support groups?

There are a number of Internet lists and newsgroups that act as online support groups for IBS (see pages 150–151). Online support groups work in a manner similar to ones that meet in person—offering shared experiences, a calming voice for the newly diagnosed, and a way to reduce the stress of living with IBS.

I'd like to go to a support group meeting, but the idea of speaking in front of groups makes me nervous. What can I do?

This is completely understandable and very common. Try talking to the facilitator ahead of time about your concerns so she doesn't single you out. Consider bringing a friend to the meeting. And don't worry if you don't talk; listening to what others have to say can be just as helpful. Take your time getting to know the people in the group. Once you feel comfortable, you'll find you have plenty to add to the discussion.

Helpful resources

American Dietetic Association
www.eatright.org
With nearly 70,000 members, the American Dietetic Association is the nation's largest organization of food and nutrition professionals.

International Foundation for Functional Gastrointestinal Disorders
www.iffgd.org

The American Gastroenterological Association
www.gastro.org

National Association of Social Workers
www.socialworkers.org

National Mental Health Association
www.nmha.org

CHAPTER 4

Treatments for IBS

Your treatment plan 64

The elimination diet 66

Over-the-counter relief 68

Probiotics 70

The brain/gut connection 72

Prescriptions for symptom relief 74

Cutting-edge drugs for IBS 76

Sleep medications 78

Psychological therapy 80

Helpful resources 82

Your treatment plan

you can create one yourself

What you eat, the kind of stress you're under, and other physical illnesses can all affect the course of your IBS on a day-to-day basis. Thus there is no one treatment regimen for IBS; typically, various treatments are required, such as medication, stress reduction, and probiotics. Moreover, the success of a treatment plan takes time. Most doctors start by tackling your diet and lifestyle issues, then consider more treatment options if those don't work. A typical protocol for treating IBS looks something like this.

Step 1. Review your diet. Discuss adding fiber to diet and cutting back on stomach irritants such as cafffeine and alcohol. For more on diet, see Chapter 6.

Step 2. Analyze the role of stress in IBS. Look to improve sleep, exercise, and diet. Consider various stress reducers such as psychotherapy or biofeedback to help combat adverse reactions to stress. For more on this, see Chapter 10.

Step 3. Treat IBS symptoms with over-the-counter medicine.

Step 4. Treat IBS symptoms with prescription medications.

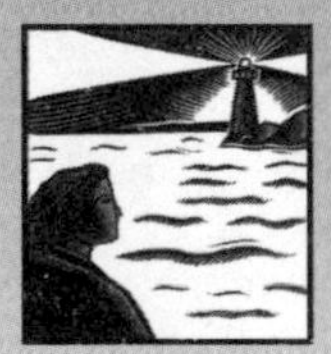

FIRST PERSON INSIGHTS

Pain—the worst part of IBS

For me, the worst part of my IBS has been the pain. Sometimes it's just a dull ache in my gut, and aspirin or Ibuprofen can keep it under control. Other times, I just lie in bed with a heating pad on my stomach, woozy from the antispasmodic pills my doctor gave me. Over the years, I've learned a lot about pain—most important is that it's subjective. I've learned that just because I hurt doesn't mean I'm weak or a whiner. And I don't let anyone else denigrate my pain or tell me that since they can't "find" anything wrong, I shouldn't be hurting. I hurt, and I deserve relief.

—Sally M., Santa Rosa, CA

Pain-Care Bill of Rights

According to the American Pain Foundation (see Helpful Resources for contact information), as a person with pain you have the right to

- Have your report of pain taken seriously and treated with dignity and respect by doctors, nurses, pharmacists, and other health care professionals.
- Have your pain thoroughly assessed and promptly treated.
- Be informed about what may be causing your pain, possible treatments, and the benefits, risks, and costs of each.
- Actively participate in decisions about how to manage your pain.
- Have your pain reassessed regularly and your treatment adjusted if your pain continues.
- Be referred to a pain specialist if your pain persists.
- Get clear and prompt answers to your questions, take time to make decisions, and refuse a particular type of treatment if you choose.

Pain Factors

These things can make your pain feel worse:

- Stress
- Overdoing physical activity
- Depression
- Anxiety
- Fatigue
- Focusing on pain

These things can help block pain signals:

- Humor
- Distraction
- Massage
- Medication
- Relaxation
- Appropriate exercise
- Heat and cold treatments

The elimination diet

if a certain food is the culprit

As you probably know by now, what you eat is intimately involved with your IBS symptoms. Perhaps you are beginning to sense that your stomach pain comes on after a breakfast of cereal and milk, but you have no problems if you have scrambled eggs. Could you have a problem with the gluten in the cereal or the lactose in the milk? How do you find out? If you or your doctor suspect that certain foods are causing or exacerbating your IBS, then you need to consider an elimination diet as part of your treatment plan.

The standard elimination diet calls for you to avoid one specific food from your diet for one to two weeks, while you keep track of your symptoms in a food diary. (See pages 98–99 for information about how to keep a food diary.) After that one-to-two-week trial is over, you then reintroduce the food into your diet and see if you experience any problems.

What foods should you eliminate first? The common culprits behind IBS seem to be gluten (a food found in wheat), lactose (the sugar found in milk), and fructose (the sugar found in fruit). Most doctors suggest starting by eliminating wheat-based products and moving on down the list. Note: Elimination diets call for keen observation skills. There is no point in following an elimination diet if you don't keep careful records of what you eat, as well as where and when, not to mention how you feel after eating.

Another option is to consider a core diet for a few weeks and then introduce new foods into your diet one week at a time. A very restricted core diet consists of bottled water, rice, and broiled meat. Very few people are allergic to these three simple foods. Or you might try eliminating all the foods you think could be causing a problem and then introducing them back into your diet one at a time.

Food That Can Trigger IBS

Alcohol and vinegar
Red wine, champagne, beer, dark-colored liquors; balsamic or red wine vinegar

Aspartame (NutraSweet)

Sorbitol
Any foods that contain this commercial sweetener

Wheat products
Bread, some cereals

Caffeine-containing beverages and foods
Regular coffee, tea, iced tea, and cola; caffeine-containing soft drinks; chocolate

Dairy products
Milk, cheese, yogurt, sour cream, and dairy-containing foods such as pizza, ice-cream bars, etc.

Fruits
Citrus fruits (oranges, grapefruit, lemons, limes) and their juices; raisins and other dried fruit; bananas, red plums, canned figs, avocados

Monsodium glutamate (MSG)
Any foods that contain MSG. Check labels of prepared foods as well as condiments to see if they contain this flavor enhancer

Snack foods and prepared foods
Hydrolyzed vegetable/soy/plant protein; natural flavorings; yeast extract; many soups, broths, and snacks

Nuts and peanut butter
All nuts and nut butters, including peanut butter

Processed meats
Hot dogs, sausage, bacon, salami, bologna, and other meats that are aged, canned, cured, marinated, tenderized, or contain nitrates

Vegetables
Broad, lima, fava, and navy beans; pea pods, sauerkraut, onions

Over-the-counter relief

laxatives and fiber supplements

Before you move on to the big guns of prescription drugs, consider these over-the-counter remedies.

Long-term relief

Fiber supplements. Although you need to increase the amount of fiber in your diet (see pages 100–101), it's nearly impossible to get the high amount of fiber you need from your diet alone (at least another 25 grams of fiber a day). That's where fiber supplements come in. They are available as powder or pills. They can be taken on a daily basis.

Short-term relief

These over-the-counter remedies should not be used daily for prolonged periods without first talking with your doctor:

Antacids and antigas medications. These medications, which carry such recognizable names as Rolaids, Tums, and Mylanta, can provide some short-term relief, particularly if you have embarrassing flatulence. But if you've been taking them and they aren't working, stop and talk to your doctor about more powerful alternatives.

Antidiarrheals. These medications, including Imodium, contain a chemical called loperamide. Some studies find they can reduce diarrhea, the urge to defecate, and abdominal pain in IBS patients.

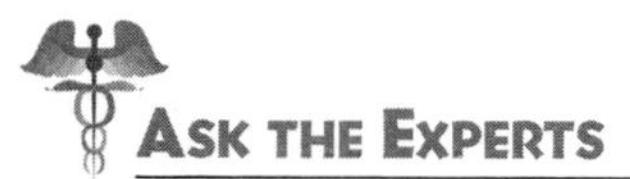

Ask the Experts

What is the best way to take fiber supplements?

Most fiber supplements are in powder form that you measure out by the teaspoon and mix with a large glass of water or juice. If you are adding fiber supplements to your diet for the first time, start with one teaspoon a day, slowly increasing the amount by teaspoons until you reach two tablespoons twice a day (in a large glass of juice or water). Going slowly will help reduce the amount of gas and bloating you'll feel as your body gets used to the extra fiber. Don't stop taking the supplement if you begin to have gas; the primary reason fiber supplements don't work is not the supplements themselves, but the fact that patients stop taking them before they have a chance to work. If you're feeling uncomfortable digestive problems after you start taking the fiber, cut back on how much you're taking and increase the amount more slowly. Also make sure you buy a supplement that contains psyllium husk, a natural, soluble plant fiber that works best for those with IBS. You can also take fiber supplements in tablet form or as a wafer. If you do that, make sure you drink a large glass of water (at least 10 ounces) with them.

Should I take over-the-counter laxatives if I'm constipated?

There is really no good evidence that laxatives, particularly those that work by absorbing water, provide any benefit to patients with IBS. In fact, some studies suggest they may actually make your bloating and gas worse. Stimulant laxatives, which irritate the intestinal wall to stimulate intense intestinal contractions, result in abdominal cramping, something you definitely can do without! Better to add small incremental amounts of fiber supplement to your diet. It may take a few days before you feel the fiber is working.

Probiotics

getting the good microorganisms

If you've ever eaten live cultured yogurt, then you've eaten **probiotics**—live bacteria that improve the overall balance of microorganisms in your digestive tract. These bacteria are found in fermented foods such as yogurt, kefir, buttermilk, and sauerkraut. In recent years they've been included as part of treatment for everything from asthma and allergies to cancer and, you guessed it, IBS.

The few studies that have been conducted on probiotics find they significantly improve symptoms in people with IBS. In one well-designed study of 40 people with IBS, those who drank a fruit drink containing probiotics before breakfast and two hours after dinner found their abdominal pain improved in just one week.

Researchers have lots of theories about why probiotics could be a good treatment for IBS. First is the fact that we're supposed to have lots of these bacteria in our gut to begin with (the most common types are lactobacilli and bifidobacteria). But modern food processing leaves precious little of these good-guy bacteria in food. Hence, it's too easy for the bad bacteria in your gut to take over—especially after a course of antibiotics, which kill the good bacteria along with the bad.

Also, IBS often develops after food poisoning or some other gastrointestinal infection. A short course of probiotics often works wonders in wiping out nasty bugs like *E. coli*, salmonella, and shigella and their toxins.

Probiotic microorganisms also generate an enzyme called nitric oxide that is thought to help the large and small intestines move food through at a normal pace, thus reducing constipation, diarrhea, and stomach pain.

Picking the Right Probiotic

But what if you hate yogurt? These days, you can get probiotics in pill form. But before you try the pills, consider a drinkable yogurt that tastes like a milk shake without the ice cream, such as Dannon's Actimel (said to be more popular in Spain than Coke). The drink contains probiotics with significantly higher bacteria counts than those in regular yogurt, as well as healthy nutrients such as calcium and protein that pill supplements don't.

When choosing a probiotic, make sure the label contains such common bacteria as *L. acidophilus, S. thermophilus, L. bulgaricus, L. casei, L. reuteri,* and/or *Bifidus.*

Living Without Dairy

If eating ice cream gives you gas and drinking milk makes you run to the bathroom, then you may be lactose intolerant in addition to having IBS. This means you lack the enzyme **lactase** needed to digest the sugar molecule **lactose** found in dairy products. Some studies find that people with IBS are more likely to be lactose intolerant than people without the condition. This doesn't mean swearing off of banana splits and double-cheese pizza forever, though. You can buy over-the-counter lactase enzymes (called Lactaid) in most drugstores. Take as directed before you reach for the ice-cream cone or order the Philly cheese steak and you should see significant relief. Lactose intolerance is fairly common in Asian, East Indian, and African-American populations. About one in three African-Americans is lactose intolerant.

The brain/gut connection

using antidepressants to overcome IBS

For years, people complaining of symptoms associated with IBS were told it was "all in their head." Even today, instead of receiving a diagnosis of IBS and appropriate treatment, many are told they simply have to relax and their symptoms will go away. While it is true that stress-reduction techniques can make a big difference in coping with IBS (more on that in Chapter 10), the bottom line is that stress does not cause IBS. It can, however, stir up an already irritated bowel. How so? Researchers think that it has something to do with the specialized communication circuits between the brain and the gut. One shared communication system involves hormones. Like the brain, the gut has receptors for various hormones, including the sex hormones, androgen, estrogen, and progesterone. These hormones trigger the intestinal muscles to contract, or they send in digestive enzymes or tell the bowel to calm down. When these hormones fluctuate, which they normally do during a woman's monthly cycle or in response to stress, they can bring on IBS symptoms. (For more on this, see pages 118–119.)

Researchers are also looking at the connections between the **central nervous system** (CNS) and the nervous system of the gastrointestinal tract, known as the **enteric nervous system,** or the **ENS**. While much of your CNS is under your conscious control, your ENS is not. It autonomically controls blood flow, smooth muscle contraction in the gut, and the movement of fluids, among other things. Both the CNS and ENS rely on neurotransmitters or chemicals to convey messages between neurons and nerves. In the brain, these messengers affect mood, pain and sleep, to name just a few. An imbalance of the neurotransmitters serotonin and dopamine can cause depression. To treat that, doctors may prescribe tricyclic antidepressants, such as Elavil and Tofranil. Serendipitously, doctors found that some of their depressed patients who had IBS got relief from both their depression and their IBS symptoms while taking tricyclics.

This prompted researchers to investigate the relationship between the brain's messengers and those found in the gut. Researchers know that the release of serotonin in the guts starts the digestive process. They surmise that IBS could be due to low levels of serotonin in the gut, which somehow offsets the digestive process, perhaps causing problems in motility. If this is true, then one way to counter that problem is to treat IBS with antidepressants that affect nerve messengers in both the brain and the gut. Studies have shown that tricyclic antidepressants have proven effective against IBS. They work by inhibiting the brain's breakdown of the neurotransmitters serotonin and norepinephrine, as well as affecting stress hormones like acetylcholine. Newer antidepressants, known as Selective Serotonin Reuptake Inhibitors (SSRIs), have also been prescribed to treat IBS. They have proven effective in some cases and have fewer side effects than tricyclics. The brain/gut connection may explain why some people with chronic IBS also have chronic depression. For those with clinical depression and IBS, they will most likely be treated with SSRIs.

Common Antidepressants for Irritable Bowel Medication

Drug Type	Generic Name (examples)	Brand Name	Potential Side Effects
Tricyclic antidepressants	Amitriptyline Desipramine Doxepin Imipramine	Elavil Norpramin Sinequan Tofranil	Sedation, weight gain, dry mouth, blurred vision, headache
SSRIs (selective serotonin reuptake inhibitors)	Citalopram Fluoxetine Fluvoxamine Paroxetine Sertraline	Celexa/Lexapro Prozac Luvox Paxil Zoloft	Some short-term nausea, reduction of libido, sleep disruption, diarrhea

Prescriptions for symptom relief
but beware the side effects

Here are some of the typical prescription medications your doctor may prescribe to relieve your symptoms.

Antispasmodics and anticholinergics. These drugs relax smooth muscle, reducing the stomach cramps and pain that are so much a part of IBS. Pain is a key part of IBS. Some researchers theorize that people with IBS are more sensitive to pain than those without IBS.

Antidiarrheals. These drugs help with diarrhea-predominant IBS.

Serotonin (5-HT4) agonists. This class of drugs works to affect the level of serotonin in the gut. Trademark drugs of this type include Zelnorm and Lotronex. The first in this class, Lotronex (alosetron), was initially approved in 2000 for diarrhea-predominant IBS but was then taken off the market because of significant side effects, including constipation complications and an inflammation of the colon called **ischemic colitis**. In 2002, the Food and Drug Administration (FDA) allowed it back on the market but severely restricted its use, limiting it to women with severe diarrhea-predominant IBS whose IBS symptoms have failed to respond to conventional therapy, and requiring patients and doctors to sign several consent forms in order to fill a prescription. Another drug in this class, called tegaserod (sold under the brand name Zelnorm) has been approved for women with constipation-predominant IBS. It does not require special consent and is well tolerated, with few side effects.

Irritable Bowel Syndrome Medications

Drug Type (examples)	Generic Name	Brand Name	Best Used For	Potential Side Effects
Antispasmodics and anticholinergics	Belladonna/ phenobarbital Dicyclomine Hyoscyamine Propantheline	Donnatal Bentylol/Bentyl Levbid/Levsin Pro-Banthine	Abdominal pain	Constipation (less common with hyoscyamine); decreased sweating; dryness of mouth, nose, throat, or skin
Antidiarrheal	Diphenoxylate/ atropine	Lomotil	Diarrhea	May become habit forming if taken over long periods of time. Side effects rare when used for short periods of time.
	Cholestyramine	Questran	Diarrhea	Constipation
Serotonin receptor agonists and antagonists	Alosetron	Lotronex	Diarrhea-predominant IBS	Approved for women only; may cause constipation or, in rare cases, colitis
	Tegaserod	Zelnorm	Constipation-predominant IBS and abdominal pain	Approved for women only

Cutting-edge drugs for IBS

better symptom relief

Ever since the first drugs specifically designed to treat IBS were introduced in 2000, pharmaceutical and biotech companies around the world have been racing to see who can bring the next—and better—IBS treatment to the market.

There is no shortage of compounds to try. Many, in fact, are in late-stage trials and may be approved within the next two to three years. Among them are the following.

Fedotozine. This drug changes the way the brain perceives sensations from the gut. In clinical trials it reduced participants' perceptions of bloating and relieved their abdominal pain.

Octreotide. Some studies suggest that this drug, sold under the brand name Sandostatin, may help in the treatment of IBS, although it's not clear exactly how it works. It seems to accelerate the movement of food through the intestine and improve bowel movements.

Muscarinic receptor antagonists. This class of drugs, which includes darifenacin and zamifenacin, helps soothe painful intestinal spasms without the adverse effects other antispasmodics may have.

Cholecystokinin (CCK) receptor antagonists. These drugs, which include the chemical loxiglumide, help food move through the gut faster, increasing bowel movement frequency and providing relief for those with constipation-predominant IBS.

Calcium channel blockers (CCBs). This class of compounds, which includes pinaverium, relaxes the smooth muscle of the gut and slows the movement of food through the digestive system, thus providing benefits for those with diarrhea-predominant IBS.

Phenylethamines. This class of drugs, which includes the experimental compound mebeverine, reduces stool frequency.

Ammonium derivatives. This class of compounds, which includes otilonium, reduces intestinal smooth-muscle movement, thus decreasing pain.

These are just a few of the new directions researchers are exploring. A good way to stay up-to-date on new therapies is through the bulletin boards and news sections of IBS Web sites, many of which can be found in Chapter 9.

Sleep medications

. . . and lifestyle changes

The connection between irritable bowel syndrome and sleep runs both ways. Not only can IBS interfere with a good night's sleep, but poor sleep can worsen your IBS symptoms. Researchers from the University of Washington in Seattle conducted a study of some 120 women (83 of whom had IBS and 35 of whom did not). The researchers wanted to test how sleep affected digestion. They asked the women to keep a diary of their sleep habits and digestion symptoms for five weeks. The researchers found that the worse night's sleep the women got, the greater their gastrointestinal symptoms the next day. This was true for both groups. Researchers aren't sure just why a bad night makes IBS symptoms so much worse, but they suspect there may be some kind of disturbance related to the central nervous system and the enteric nervous system that affects both sleep and gastrointestinal disorders. Serotonin, the neurotransmitter that regulates your body's ability to control pain and mood, also facilitates deep, restorative sleep. Some experts believe that levels of serotonin may be low or poorly processed in IBS patients—thus the poor sleep patterns.

There are several lifestyle changes you can make to improve your ability to fall and stay asleep. However, if you are really having difficulty getting your sleep back on track, ask your doctor about a short-term use of prescription medication. Today's new sleep aids are much less likely to leave you with a sleep "hangover" than the drugs of years before, nor are they likely to become addicting. Like any medication, prescription sleep aids do have side effects, such as dizziness and headaches.

If you choose to use over-the-counter sleep aids, be aware that most of them contain antihistamines—medicine that is commonly found in over-the-counter allergy medications. Side effects include constipation, dry mouth, anxiety, and possible "rebound" insomnia once you stop taking them.

Getting a good night's sleep

- Avoid napping during the day if you're having trouble sleeping at night.
- Avoid vigorous exercise in the evening.
- If you are taking diuretics (water pills), don't take them at bedtime; this will save you from needing to urinate during the night.
- Stay away from large meals close to bedtime.
- Avoid any caffeine (coffee, colas, and chocolate) after 4 p.m.
- Establish a regular relaxing bedtime routine. Avoid emotionally upsetting conversations and activities before trying to go to sleep.
- Make sure your sleep environment is pleasant and relaxing. The bed should be comfortable; the room should not be too hot or cold, or too bright.
- Don't spend too much time in bed. If you have trouble falling asleep, get up for a while, then try again. Use your bed only for sex and sleep.

Sleep Medication

Drug Type	Generic Name (examples)	Brand Name	Potential Side Effects
Benzo-diazepines	Estazolam Flurazepam Quazepam Temazepam Triazolam	ProSom Dalmane Doral Restoril Halcion	Stomach upset, headache, depression, dizziness, memory impairment, next-day hangover; potential for abuse/addiction
Nonbenzo-diazepine, benzodi-azepine receptor agonists	Zaleplon Zolpidem	Sonata Ambien	Dizziness, heart palpitations, amnesia, headache, rash
Sedating anti-depressants	Amitriptyline Doxepin Trazodone	Elavil Sinequan Desyrel	Dry mouth, headache, increased appetite, unpleasant taste, weight gain, urinary retention

Psychological therapy

certain talk therapies can really help

Maybe you think your IBS is "all in your head" and that if you were only stronger, you could "get over it." This kind of thinking is not only depressing, but it could make your symptoms worse by increasing your own stress. One therapy shown in numerous studies to help with IBS is cognitive-behavioral therapy, or CBT. This is a form of short-term psychotherapy lasting about 12 weeks that emphasizes the vital role your thinking plays in how you interpret events and feelings.

For instance, through CBT you can learn that IBS is indeed a medical disorder, one that is still relatively mysterious in terms of its causes but that is physical in nature. When thoughts such as "this is all in my head" arise, you can replace them with ones you learn in CBT, such as "IBS is a genuine physical disorder."

Or maybe you view the pain that often accompanies IBS as something that is your fault or a sign you have failed in your treatment. A CBT-trained therapist can help you learn to view your pain not as a failing but as a signal to slow down, to take it easy, to rest.

Through CBT, you can learn how to change the way you react to problematic or stressful situations. For instance, if you notice through your symptom diary that you often have IBS symptoms after a visit with your sister, a CBT therapist can help you identify ways to cope better with your sister without becoming upset. Overall, your CBT therapist should provide information about IBS and normal gastrointestinal functioning, help you identify triggers that make your symptoms worse, teach you relaxation techniques (some of which are described on pages 166–167), help you identify and replace irrational thoughts regarding your problems (e.g., "I can never go on vacation again"), and help you find ways to manage some of the more uncomfortable social situations that may arise with IBS.

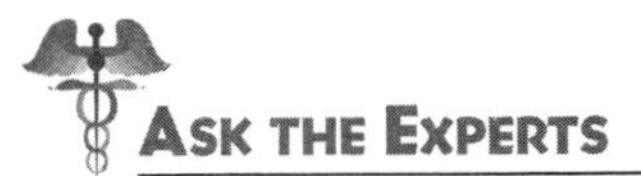

Ask the Experts

What is the difference between cognitive-behavioral therapy (CBT) and psychoanalysis or "talk" therapy?

One major difference is the amount of time required. CBT generally takes an average of 12 sessions to see significant results, while traditional talk therapy can take years. One reason for the difference is that CBT focuses on specific incidents and concerns in your life, rather than trying to unravel every facet of your life from your childhood to the present. Also, during CBT you must complete homework assignments. This helps you to change the way you view events and think about things, like your illness, much more quickly.

Where can I find a therapist who knows cognitive-behavioral therapy?

You can contact the National Association of Cognitive-Behavioral Therapists at 800-853-1135 or scan the group's Web site for a listing of therapists near you at **www.nacbt.org**.

Helpful resources

A Victim No More: Overcoming Irritable Bowel Syndrome
by Jonathan M. Berkowitz, M.D.

Irritable Bowel Syndrome
by Sarah Brewer, M.D.

The Chronic Pain Solution
by James N. Dillard, M.D.

Relief from IBS
by Elaine Fantle Shimberg

The Second Brain: A Groundbreaking New Understanding of Nervous Disorders of the Stomach and Intestines
by Michael D. Gershon, M.D.

IBS: A Doctor's Plan for Chronic Digestive Troubles
by Gerard Guillory, M.D.

Listen to Your Gut
by Jini Patel Thompson

American Pain Foundation
888-615-7246

American Chronic Pain Association
916-632-0922
www.theacpa.org

National Association of Cognitive-Behavioral Therapists
800-853-1135
www.nacbt.org

Chapter 5

Overlapping Syndromes

Fibromyalgia 84

Chronic fatigue syndrome 86

Interstitial cystitis 88

Migraine 90

Chronic pelvic pain 92

Helpful resources 94

Fibromyalgia

striking similarities

It is estimated that up to 50 percent of people with **fibromyalgia** (a complex pain disorder) also have IBS. Like IBS, fibromyalgia is a functional disorder, meaning that for now there is no known organic cause. Nor are there any definitive medical tests to determine whether you have fibromyalgia. Once your doctor has ruled out other disorders, he must look to your pain symptoms to guide him toward a diagnosis of fibromyalgia. Fibromyalgia is usually diagnosed when you have specific tender points in all four quadrants of your body for at least three months. This means you have muscle pain on both the right and left sides of your body, as well as above and below your waist and down your spine. All together, there are 18 designated tender points at which you might feel pain when pressure is applied, including your knees, buttocks, hips, neck and shoulders, and chest. If you have pain in at least 11 of those points, you may have fibromyalgia.

Another similarity between fibromyalgia and IBS is that fibromyalgia appears to be related to an increased sensitivity to pain. In fact, some researchers theorize that people with fibromyalgia may process pain differently than those without the condition. This is also considered to be a possible underlying cause of IBS, in which people with IBS process sensations in their digestive tract differently than those without the condition. Plus, pain processing is associated with serotonin, the neurotransmitter that plays a big role in the digestive system (for more on serotonin see pages 72–73).

Common Fibromyalgia Symptoms

The following are common physical and emotional symptoms of fibromyalgia. Note how many are similar to the symptoms of IBS described on pages 16–17.

Physical symptoms

- Fatigue
- Muscle tenderness
- Sleep disturbance
- Pain all over
- Joint pain and tenderness
- Morning stiffness
- Numbness and tingling in arms, legs, feet, or face
- Feeling cold
- Night sweats
- Changes in bowel habits
- Migraine headaches
- Dry, itchy eyes
- Jaw pain
- Chest pain or tightness
- Feeling of swollen joints
- Abdominal cramps

Emotional symptoms

- Noticeable anxiety and excitability
- Mood swings, including bouts of crying
- Irritability and impatience
- Impaired memory
- Slowing of mental processes
- Inability to concentrate
- Loss of interest in normal activities
- Confused thinking
- Depression
- Loss of interest in sex
- Withdrawal from friends and family

Chronic fatigue syndrome

enduring exhaustion

One of the most common symptoms of IBS is fatigue. This could be related simply to the wearing nature of the condition, or it could be a sign of another overlapping syndrome, **chronic fatigue syndrome**, or CFS. More than half of those with IBS are also diagnosed with CFS. Note: Fatigue could also be a sign of clinical depression.

Chronic fatigue syndrome is marked by clinical fatigue (lasting longer than six months), sleep problems, concentration and short-term memory problems, sore throat, low-grade fevers, headaches, and tender lymph nodes. As with IBS, there is no known organic cause, although researchers suspect that a flulike virus or injury may trigger its onset. Often people with CFS report that their symptoms began after they contracted a cold, bronchitis, hepatitis, mononucleosis, or an intestinal bug. Not coincidentally, IBS often develops after an extreme bout of gastroenteritis, or stomach upset caused by a bacteria or virus.

Although studies find that about half of those with CFS recover, most within five years, some get progressively worse while others alternate between periods of illness and comparative well-being.

As with IBS, there is no definitive diagnostic blood test to determine whether you have CFS. Instead, your doctor will ask you a series of questions to rule out other conditions. While there is no cure as yet for CFS, various treatments can help with symptom management, such as nonsteroidal anti-inflammatory drugs (NSAIDs) like Advil or Motrin.

Longer-term treatments for CFS mimic many for IBS, including eating a balanced diet, getting lots of rest, exercising regularly, and avoiding and managing stress. Doctors may also prescribe antidepressants (see pages 72–73).

Dysregulation Spectrum Syndrome

The similarities between conditions like fibromyalgia, chronic fatigue syndrome, and IBS have spawned a theory that such disorders, which also include migraine, restless legs syndrome (RLS), and pain during menstrual periods, may be related. The theory comes from Muhammad Yunus, M.D., a fibromyalgia researcher. He groups the conditions together and calls them **dysregulation spectrum syndrome.** The symptoms of this syndrome, he says, are related to abnormal secretions from glands and the nervous system, essentially putting the nervous system on high alert and increasing the perception of certain sensations, such as pain and digestive distress.

Symptoms of chronic fatigue syndrome

- Noticeable anxiety and excitability
- Recurrent low-grade fever
- Irritability and impatience
- Impaired memory
- Inability to concentrate
- Loss of interest in normal activities
- Problems sleeping
- Depression
- Loss of interest in sex
- Withdrawal from friends and family

Interstitial cystitis

a sudden urge to go

People with IBS, particularly women, often find they experience not only the bowel-related problems of IBS such as diarrhea and constipation but urinary-related symptoms as well. These include a strong and sudden urge to urinate, frequent urination (more than every two hours), waking up in the middle of the night to urinate, and the sense that they haven't completely emptied their bladder. Add chronic urinary pain to the mix and you have a recipe for interstitial cystitis.

Interstitial cystitis, or IC, is a chronic inflammatory condition of the bladder. It is not related to "common" cystitis, or urinary tract infections, which can be cured with antibiotics. Interstitial cystitis affects about 700,000 women in the United States, although it can also occur in men. In one major study of women with IC, one in three of these women were found to also have IBS. As with many conditions that overlap with IBS, interstitial cystitis worsens under stressful situations, although it is not caused by stress. There is also no specific test for it. To determine a diagnosis, your doctor will take urine cultures to rule out a bacterial infection and conduct urinary tests such as a cystoscopy or biopsy of the bladder to rule out bladder cancer, kidney problems, vaginal infections, and other conditions. During a cystoscopy, you are put to sleep and the doctor uses a thin telescopelike instrument fitted with a light and camera to view the inside of your bladder.

Although there is no cure for interstitial cystitis, there are several treatments for its symptoms, ranging from medications such as Elmiron (pentosan), the only drug approved specifically for IC, to the same medications used to treat IBS, including tricyclic antidepressants, anti-inflammatory agents, and antispasmodics. Doctors also suggest making certain lifestyle changes, such as eliminating certain spicy and acidic foods, stopping smoking, cutting out coffee, tea, and alcohol, and reducing stress.

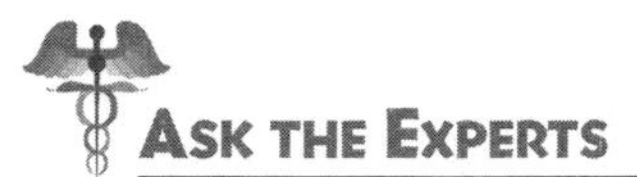

Ask the Experts

I've heard about something called electronic nerve stimulation to treat interstitial cystitis. What is it and does it work?

Transcutaneous electrical nerve stimulation, or TENS, is a pain relief system that uses a special device to transmit electrical impulses through electrodes into the painful part of the body. While it doesn't cure the pain, it does block it, providing some temporary relief. TENS sessions last between 10 minutes and two hours, and for those with IC, daily sessions of at least 30 minutes are recommended.

Other electrical stimulating devices being tested on people with IC include neuromodulation, which uses electrical stimulation to influence nerve activity through the spinal cord, and sacral nerve stimulation implants, which are surgically implanted into the part of the spine known as the sacral nerve roots that helps control sensation in the urinary tract.

Symptoms of interstitial cystitis syndrome

- Frequent urination during the day and evening, up to 60 times a day in some cases
- The feeling that you have to urinate immediately, which may also be accompanied by pain, pressure, or spasms
- Pain in the lower abdominal, urethral, or vaginal area
- Pain with sexual intercourse
- Painful muscles and joints
- Migraines

Migraine

all in your head

Migraine headaches affect 28 million Americans, 75 percent of them women. They are also closely linked to IBS, with several studies finding that people with IBS are highly susceptible to migraines.

Researchers suspect several reasons behind the connection. One is related to a condition known as abdominal migraine, often diagnosed in children, in which some underlying inflammatory lesion in the digestive area causes headaches. There are also connections between diet and migraine just as there are between diet and IBS. For instance, people with migraine are cautioned to keep away from certain foods, such as aged cheese, chocolate, and red wine, known to trigger the devastating headaches.

Migraines are known to be a condition of the **neurovascular system**, meaning that the entire nervous system, including the brain and the spinal cord and your blood vessels—are all involved in the process. An over- or underactive neurovascular system may also be responsible for IBS.

Plus, there is a wide overlap between neurotransmitters in the digestive system, such as serotonin, and those in the brain. One theory suggests that when someone who is susceptible to migraines encounters a trigger, such as food, light, or stress, it causes changes in the levels of chemical signalers in the brain, specifically serotonin and noradrenalin, the same chemicals involved in IBS, resulting in a migraine headache.

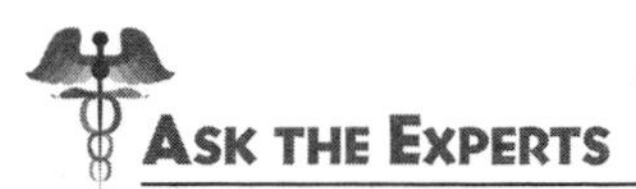

Ask the Experts

How do I know if my headache is tension or migraine?

A tension headache is most likely due to tension in the neck and scalp muscles. These muscles often contract during intense activity or stressful situations, producing pressurelike pain on both sides of your head. But a migraine typically occurs on just one side of the head, often with a throbbing feeling. Unlike with a tension headache, it is difficult to function with a migraine, which may take hours or even days to improve. Migraines are also often accompanied by nausea, vomiting, weakness, irritability, dizziness, and sensitivity to light. Some people also experience auras, or warning signs, with migraines, such as a particular smell. (Because first-time migraine symptoms can be signs of certain neurological disorders, it is important to have your migraine evaluated by a doctor.)

Is there any cure for migraine?

So far, medication can provide only symptom relief, interrupting migraines in process or reducing their frequency. Many people with migraine find relief in over-the-counter or prescription medication and in complementary therapies such as acupuncture or biofeedback. Additionally, certain medications, such as antidepressants and betablockers can, when taken prophylactically (in other words, when you don't have a migraine), help prevent frequent migraines.

Chronic pelvic pain

interfering with daily life

Although the true incidence of **chronic pelvic pain**, or CPP, is unknown, it is estimated to affect an estimated one in seven women—and half of all women with irritable bowel syndrome. Sometimes called a headache in the pelvis, CPP is marked by constant pain in the pelvic region lasting at least six months and unrelated to menstruation or any specific cause.

Just as with IBS, women with CPP were once told their pain was "all in their heads." But today physicians recognize CPP as a real functional disorder, one that sends about one in four affected women to bed an average of 2.6 days a month and forces more than half to cut down on their usual activities one or more days a month. Estimates put the incidence of CPP at nearly 9.2 million women.

Six features are common to those with chronic pelvic pain syndrome:

- The pain has been present for six months or more.
- Conventional treatments haven't helped.
- Even if some tissue damage has occurred, the level of pain is much higher than might be expected.
- There are signs of depression, including problems sleeping and diminished appetite.
- Physical activity is limited.
- Roles in the family are altered as the person with CPP becomes unable to cope with day-to-day activities.

Before making a diagnosis of CPP, your doctor will likely conduct a multitude of tests to rule out numerous other diseases and conditions that can cause pelvic pain, such as endometriosis, sexually transmitted diseases, interstitial cystitis, and vulvar disorders, such as **vulvar vestibulitis**. Women with this condition have severe sensitivity to touch at their vaginal opening and experience pain after sexual intercourse.

Treating Chronic Pelvic Pain Syndrome

As with any functional disorder, treatment for chronic pelvic pain syndrome relies on numerous approaches. In addition to pain medication, physical therapy is an integral part of any treatment program. Therapy includes exercises to stretch or strengthen certain muscles. Other treatments include transcutaneous electrical nerve stimulation (TENS), biofeedback, relaxation and breathing exercises, and psychological counseling.

Typical symptoms of chronic pelvic pain syndrome

- Anxiety and depression
- Involuntary contractions (spasms) of the muscles in the pelvic area
- Mental and physical fatigue
- Rectal itching
- Burning during frequent bowel movements
- Sleep interruptions
- Lower back pain and a feeling of heaviness in the lower abdomen
- Leg pain that radiates from the groin
- Constipation or diarrhea
- Irregular or painful menstrual cycles

Helpful resources

Barnes & Noble Health Basics: Migraine
by Joan Raymond

Heal Your Headache:
The 1-2-3 Program for
Taking Charge of Your Pain
by David Buchholz and Stephen G. Reich

Conquering Chronic Fatigue:
Answers to America's Most
Misunderstood Epidemic
by Jonathan Forester

The Interstitial Cystitis Survival Guide:
Your Guide to the Latest Treatment
Options and Coping Strategies
by Robert M. Moldwin

Chronic Fatigue and Immune
Dysfunction Syndrome
www.cfids.org

Fibromyalgia Community
www.fibrohugs.com

Interstitial Cystitis Network
www.ic-network.com

The International Pelvic Pain Society
www.pelvicpain.org

The National Migraine Association
(MAGNUM)
A national nonprofit group that acts
as a clearinghouse for information
about migraines.
www.migraines.org

Chapter 6

The Role of Nutrition and Exercise

Food fundamentals 96

A food diary 98

Fiber and IBS 100

The fructose question 102

The role of fat in IBS 104

Food intolerances 106

What about alcohol? 108

Reading food labels 110

Eating right 112

Exercise and IBS 114

Helpful resources 116

Food fundamentals

what does food have to do with IBS? plenty

You just came home from a lovely dinner out with your husband. He had the fish, you had the beef. He had a side of asparagus, you had french fries. He had sorbet for dessert, you had chocolate cake. And now you're in the bathroom, feeling like your insides are being ripped out, bemoaning the fact that you ate at all, and promising yourself that from now on, you're going to subsist on bread and water alone.

Hold on. While it's true that diet plays a major role in IBS symptoms and episodes, it's also true that you can design an IBS-friendly diet that doesn't have you living without the plethora of wonderful foods available today. The key, as with everything in life, is learning what works and doesn't work for you, and then maintaining moderation.

Unfortunately, there are no set dietary guidelines for people with IBS, and what works for one person might not work for another. Conversely, what sends your friend with IBS running to the bathroom may not even trigger a belch in you. One food may cause an IBS attack one day; two weeks later, when you timidly try that same food again, nothing.

Yes, it's infuriating. But no, it isn't unsolvable, and years of trial and error have turned up some common food enemies. Through the use of a food diary and an elimination diet and by paying close attention to what your body is trying to tell you, you can not only reduce your IBS symptoms but improve your overall health with a more nutritious diet.

Smart IBS eating tips

In addition to the dietary advice you will read throughout this chapter, there are things you can do around eating that may help with your IBS symptoms. These include:

◆ **Eat small meals more frequently.** Every time you eat, your colon contracts. Smaller meals eaten more often, or even just smaller portions, can reduce contractions, thus reducing pain and symptoms.

◆ **Eat slowly and in a serene environment.** Don't talk about anything stressful or upsetting while you're eating, which, as you know, can make your symptoms worse.

◆ **Drink lukewarm beverages.** No one knows why this is, but drinking very hot or very cold liquids can aggravate your IBS symptoms. Instead, drink your liquids lukewarm either before or after eating, not during.

◆ **Stay active after eating.** Taking a walk or working in the garden, even just washing the dishes keeps you upright and moving, which, in turn, helps your digestive system work better.

◆ **Avoid highly spiced food.** This includes curries and foods seasoned with lots of garlic, ginger, hot chili, and other peppers.

◆ **Drink at least eight 8-ounce glasses of water a day.** This helps soften stool if you're struggling with constipation and replaces lost fluid if you experience diarrhea.

A food diary

assessing where you are

Quick. What did you eat yesterday? How about the day before? Remembering everything we eat—including between-meal snacks, that bit of doughnut from your husband's breakfast, the extra fish stick you picked off your kid's plate—is about as easy as remembering the names of the 10 people you just met at a cocktail party. That's where a food diary comes in. Consider it your first step in your IBS dietary makeover, and an absolute necessity in figuring out what foods do and don't work for you.

Start by getting a small portable daily diary. In it, note down the key items on the next page. It's really important that you take your food diary with you when you leave the house, because you never know when you're going to stop for a snack.

It's important that you write down what you eat, with approximate portions, just after you finish eating—otherwise you'll forget what you ate, or how much. If you're eating alone, jot down what you're eating while you eat. If you're at a dinner party or some other public venue, do your jotting in the bathroom.

You also need to be detailed. This means writing down everything you eat—not just the steak but the ketchup you poured over it. And not just the tuna, but the two tablespoons of mayo and relish you mixed into it. Don't forget the creamer you pour in your coffee, the glass of wine you have before dinner, the soda you sip during the staff meeting, or the jam you spread on your toast. And be sure to include how quickly you ate as well as what you were doing while eating. You never know just what might be triggering your IBS symptoms, and you won't know unless you write down everything. For instance, some people find that their IBS symptoms get worse if they eat too fast. Your food journal will show if you're rushing through your meals.

My food journal

Day of the week

M T (W) T F S S

Food/drink (note amount eaten)

Breakfast

Lunch

Dinner

Snacks

What you were doing while eating

Time spent eating

Physical reaction (2 hours after eating)

Fiber and IBS

culprit and hero

Although every person with IBS is different, certain similarities in terms of what foods help and what foods hurt have come to light. One of the most important food types to learn about is fiber.

Fiber is the part of every plant food that can't be digested. There are two types of fiber: soluble and nonsoluble. The soluble type dissolves in water (think of fiber supplements like Metamucil) and is found in foods such as oat bran, barley, peas, beans, and citrus fruits. Insoluble fiber (which doesn't dissolve in water) is found in wheat bran and some vegetables. Both pass through your body undigested, acting as a kind of broom to sweep out toxins and other harmful compounds lurking in your intestines.

Soluble fiber helps your digestive system function normally. It adds bulk to your stools and absorbs water, making it easier for your body to pass stool and preventing diarrhea. That's why increasing the amount of soluble fiber is particularly important for people with both the constipation and diarrhea form of IBS.

Insoluble fiber, commonly known as roughage, can be a Catch-22 for people with IBS. In some people, this form of fiber can trigger IBS symptoms. Insoluble fiber stimulates the gastrointestinal system, speeding the passage of food through your intestines. Because you need many of the foods that contain insoluble fiber for a healthy diet, some experts suggest combining insoluble and soluble fiber—and that you never eat insoluble fiber on an empty stomach. So, for instance, you might combine a bowl of oatmeal with a fruit smoothie or eat your raw vegetables with a bowl of brown rice. Also, pureeing vegetables and fruits, as well as removing their skins, will reduce the amount of insoluble fiber you get. Keep in mind that many foods contain both soluble and insoluble fiber. For instance, a potato skin is insoluble fiber; the potato inside provides soluble fiber.

Start slow with fiber

You don't want to jump from 10 grams of fiber a day to 25 all at once. If you do, you may experience some bloating and flatulence. Instead, gradually add about 4 grams every other day, cutting back if you experience stomach problems, until you're able to handle large amounts. Four grams is about the amount of fiber found in a whole apple with skin.

Great fiber sources

Soluble fiber	Insoluble fiber
Oat bran (raw)	Wheat bran (raw)
Raspberries	Bulgur wheat
Lentils	Barley, pearled
Chick peas	Bread, whole wheat
Apples	Brown rice
Carrots	Pasta

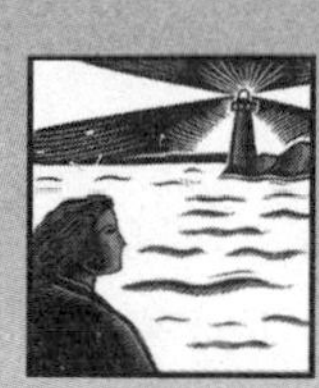

FIRST PERSON INSIGHTS

Thinking ahead

I began having diarrhea and other IBS symptoms in 1989 after a bout with gastroenteritis. Since then, my IBS sometimes renders me housebound. After much experimentation, I found my symptoms were less severe if I stuck to a rice-based, nonglutinous diet, low in fats and without spices or raw salads, and with well-cooked foods. This can make it difficult when we eat out, but if we're going to a friend's house, I often just bring something along for myself, explaining to my hostess about my "problem." Everyone so far has been so nice about it, and the hostess appreciates not having to cook a separate meal for me.

Carol K., St. Petersburg, FL

The fructose question

are fruit sugars to blame?

For several years, researchers in Iowa have been investigating how fructose, the simple sugar found in honey and many fruits, might play a role in some of the symptoms of IBS. What they've found is that fructose intolerance, or the inability of your body to tolerate fruit sugar, is present in one-third to one-half of patients with IBS symptoms. This intolerance is a genetic condition caused by the lack of a certain enzyme needed to break down fructose.

Fructose intolerance has become a major problem in the United States in the past 15 years because food manufacturers have increasingly replaced the sweetener sucrose with the sweeter and less expensive sweetener fructose. The key is to avoid products containing fructose as well as sucrose. When the Iowa researchers taught people with IBS how to eliminate fructose from their diet, their symptoms significantly decreased. Unfortunately, of 80 people participating in the study, only half actually followed the diet.

Foods to avoid if you are fructose intolerant

- Any foods with sucrose and sorbitol (see page 103)
- Any foods that list "sugar" as an ingredient
- Fruit
- Processed meats like hot dogs and cold cuts. They often contain sugar
- Fruit juices, sodas, and other drinks that contain sugars
- Mayonnaise, mustards, ketchup, marmalades, jellies, syrups, salad dressings made with sugar
- Sweetened dairy products (like fruit yogurts, ice cream, etc.)
- Sweet potatoes
- Carrots, tomatoes, corn, canned vegetables with sugar
- Most desserts
- Sugar-coated cereals
- Bread and crackers other than saltines and soda crackers

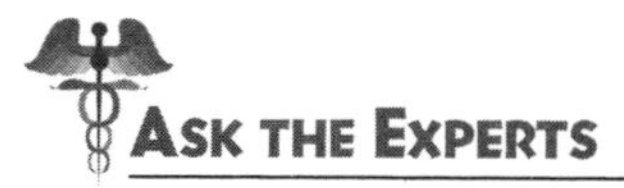

Ask the Experts

How do I find out if I'm fructose intolerant?

A simple breath test called hydrogen testing can help determine if you're fructose intolerant. Hydrogen is among the gases produced in your intestines as bacteria break down carbohydrates like fructose. Measuring the amount of hydrogen in your breath tells your doctor if your body is having a difficult time breaking down or absorbing these carbohydrates. There is also a new DNA test that can detect the hereditary form of fructose intolerance.

Are there any sugars that are okay to consume if I'm fructose intolerant?

You should be all right eating foods that contain glucose, dextrin, and maltose sweeteners. Also try the natural sweetener stevia, available in health food stores and some groceries.

My doctor told me to avoid foods with sorbitol. What's sorbitol?

Sorbitol is a sweet-tasting sugar alcohol used in many sugar-free or "dietetic" candies, cake mixes, syrups, and other foods, as well as in some medicines. It provides fewer calories than regular sugars because it is poorly absorbed by the body. However, the Center for Science in the Public Interest (CSPI), which serves as a watchdog for various nutritional issues, notes that studies over the past 15 years found that sorbitol can cause gastrointestinal symptoms ranging from mild discomfort to severe diarrhea. People with IBS tend to have effects at the more severe extreme and should probably stay away from products that use sorbitol.

The role of fat in IBS

all fats worsen the symptoms

When researchers from the Mayo Clinic Foundation in Rochester, MN, mailed a questionnaire to more than 200 Minnesotans aged 20 to 50, they found that those with IBS said they ate significantly more fat as an overall percentage of their diet than those without IBS. The results, of course, strongly suggest that a high fat intake might play a role in IBS symptoms.

All fats make IBS symptoms worse, whether it's the good fats (monounsaturated and polyunsaturated) or the bad fats (saturated and trans-fats). That's because fat acts as a stimulant to the digestive system. As the contractions of your colon increase, so, too, do the pain and other digestive symptoms of IBS.

For this reason, a low-fat diet can be a godsend for those with IBS. To follow such a diet, you have to watch out not only for traditional sources of fat (like fried foods, cakes, cookies, ice cream), but for food you might not think of as fatty, like salad dressings, mashed potatoes, hamburgers, and cheese. Luckily, today's stores are filled with hundreds of fat-free and low-fat products. Just check the labels carefully; sometimes manufacturers replace the fat with extra sugars, which can also be an IBS trigger.

What Fat-free Really Means

The U.S. Food and Drug Administration regulates all nutritional and health claims. Here's what the manufacturers' slogans really mean:

◆ **Calorie-free:** Fewer than 5 calories per serving.

◆ **Sugar-free and fat-free:** Less than 0.5 grams per serving.

◆ **Low, little, few, low source of, contains a small amount of:** Can be eaten frequently without exceeding dietary guidelines for fat, saturated fat, cholesterol, sodium, and/or calories.

◆ **Low-fat:** 3 grams or less per serving.

◆ **Low saturated fat:** 1 gram or less per serving.

◆ **Low-calorie:** 40 calories or less per serving.

◆ **Lean:** Less than 10 grams fat, 4.5 grams or less saturated fat, and less than 95 mg cholesterol per serving and per 100 grams.

◆ **Extra-lean:** Less than 5 grams of fat, less than 2 grams of saturated fat, and less than 95 mg cholesterol per serving and per 100 grams.

◆ **High:** Contains 20 percent or more of the Daily Reference Value for a particular nutrient in a serving. (See Daily Reference Value chart on page 111.)

◆ **Good source:** One serving contains 10 to 19 percent of the Daily Reference Value for a particular nutrient.

◆ **Reduced:** This nutritionally altered product contains at least 25 percent less of a nutrient or of calories than the regular version.

◆ **Less or fewer:** Means that a food, whether altered or not, contains 25 percent less of a nutrient or of calories than the regular version.

◆ **Light:** The food has one-third fewer calories or half the fat of the "reference" food, or the sodium content has been cut by 50 percent.

◆ **Healthy:** Must be low in fat and saturated fat and contain limited amounts of cholesterol and sodium, among other requirements.

Food intolerances

lactose and wheat

Lactose intolerance is a genetic trait affecting about one in 10 Caucasians, but up to six in 10 Asians (up to nine in 10 Chinese) and eight in 10 African Americans. It means you're missing an enzyme necessary to digest lactase, the sugar found in dairy products, particularly milk. So every time you have a bowl of ice cream or a cup of milk, you wind up with diarrhea, gas, and bloating—all symptoms of IBS. In fact, many people with IBS are also lactose intolerant.

Similarly, some researchers suspect that people with IBS may also be intolerant to wheat, which plays a huge role in most people's diet. In fact, estimates are that Americans eat several hundred grams per day of wheat, about 10 to 15 percent of which cannot be digested.

You can get tested for lactose and wheat intolerance, but the easiest technique is simply to eliminate them from your diet (as described on pages 66–67), then slowly add one wheat or dairy item at a time to your diet to see if the symptoms return.

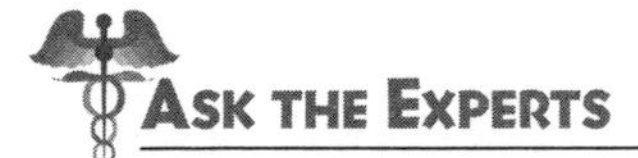

Ask the Experts

How does IBS differ from celiac disease?

Celiac disease causes a malabsorption of nutrients after you eat foods that contain gluten—protein found in wheat. It can cause diarrhea and gas and fatty, foul-smelling stools. Celiac is usually diagnosed by a biopsy of the small intestine. Unlike IBS, celiac can lead to malnutrition.

I'm worried about colon cancer because I have IBS. Is there anything I can do to reduce my risk?

First, there is no evidence that you have a higher risk of colon cancer if you have IBS. Still, there are numerous ways you can reduce your overall risk of colon cancer through a healthy diet. This includes getting plenty of fiber through your food—not through a supplement—and watching your weight (the risk of colon cancer increases if you're overweight or obese). Eating plenty of fruits and vegetables has also been shown in several studies to reduce your risk. And, if you are over 50, or younger and you have a family history of colon cancer, it is important to have a colonoscopy and fecal occult blood tests.

How do I find a dietitian?

You can find a dietitian on your own through the yellow pages or by contacting the American Dietetic Association at 800-877-1600, ext. 5000, or at **www.eatright.org.**

What is the difference between a food allergy and a food intolerance?

A food allergy implies there is an allergic, or immunologic, response when a certain food is eaten or the body is exposed to a certain allergen. A food intolerance means the body, for a variety of reasons, has difficulty digesting a certain food, but no true allergy exists.

What about alcohol?

don't overdo it

Who doesn't like a glass of wine with dinner, or a cold beer on a hot summer's afternoon? But if you have IBS, such imbibing can bring you more than a relaxed feeling. It can serve as a trigger for your symptoms. Plus, if you're taking prescription medications for your IBS, the alcohol can interact with the medication. Alcohol also puts more stress on your liver, which has to strain out toxins.

Alcohol may affect your IBS in other ways. For one, it stimulates the digestive system. Studies find that people tend to eat more when they're drinking alcohol, meaning you could become overly full. Also, the stimulatory effects of alcohol could increase the contractions of the digestive system, causing diarrhea among other problems. Plus, alcohol can affect the lining of the gastrointestinal tract, irritating it and causing nausea, vomiting, diarrhea, and bleeding (symptoms that IBS patients already have a tough time controlling).

National health guidelines call for everyone—those with and without IBS—to have no more than one alcoholic drink a day for women, and no more than two for men.

You can still enjoy social occasions without drinking alcohol (and without long explanations about your IBS) by following these tips:

- Choose seltzer water with a lime. It will look like a gin and tonic and you won't have to answer any questions about why you're not drinking.
- Tell people you're the designated driver and so must stay sober.
- Choose alcohol-free "beers" and "wines."
- Order fancy drinks without the alcohol. For instance, instead of a cosmopolitan, ask the bartender to mix some cranberry juice and seltzer water and pour it into a martini glass. Or order a virgin daiquiri.

Ask the Experts

Am I more likely to have problems with alcohol if I have IBS?

One of the few studies ever conducted on the connection between alcoholism and IBS looked at the prevalence of IBS among 31 patients seeking treatment for alcoholism compared to 40 patients seeking treatment for general medical problems in a primary care doctor's office. The researchers found that 42 percent of the patients with alcohol abuse or dependence had IBS, in contrast to 2.5 percent of the comparison group. They suspect that the higher prevalence of IBS among people with alcohol problems may be related to the fact that depression is so often found among people with IBS, and people with depression are also more likely to have alcohol problems. The researchers also noted, however, that symptoms of IBS may be mistakenly attributed to alcohol abuse, leading to underdiagnosis and undertreatment of IBS.

One alcoholic drink equals . . .

4–5 ounces of wine

10 ounces of wine cooler

12 ounces of beer

1 1/4 ounces of distilled liquor
(80 proof whiskey, vodka, scotch, or rum)

Reading food labels

know what to look out for

Anyone with any kind of digestive condition needs to learn to become an avid reader—of food labels, that is. The Food and Drug Administration requires that every packaged food—from a frozen dinner to a pack of gum—contain a comprehensive label providing a plethora of nutritional information.

Here's what to look for and how to read it.

Serving size. Important because it influences all the nutrient amounts listed on the top part of the label.

Calories and calories from fat. Not only can eating too many calories overall lead to obesity, which can make your IBS worse, but fat is a known trigger of IBS; the fewer calories from fat, the better.

Nutrients. Some you want to make sure you get enough of, like dietary fiber, vitamin A, C, calcium, and iron; others you want to limit, like fat, cholesterol, and sodium. If you're cutting out dairy, for instance, you want to make sure you're upping your intake of calcium from other foods.

Percent Daily Value (%DV). This tells you whether a serving of food contributes a lot or a little of the necessary nutrients to your total daily diet, or all the foods you eat in a day.

Ingredient list. You're looking for pseudonyms for fat and sugar, among other things. Other names for sugar include corn syrup, sorbitol, dextrose, glucose, fructose, maltose, honey, and molasses.

Ask the Experts

What is a Daily Reference Value?

Daily Reference Values (DRVs) are the amount of macronutrients (i.e., fat, protein, and carbohydrate) set by the National Academy of Sciences. They're based on the number of calories you eat every day. All labels use a basic 2,000-calorie diet as a reference point. That figure was chosen because it's the daily calorie requirement for postmenopausal women, the group with the highest risk for too many calories and too much fat.

Fat: 65 grams or less

Saturated fatty acids: 20 grams or less

Cholesterol: 300 milligrams or less

Total carbohydrates: 300 grams

Fiber: 25 grams

Sodium: 2,400 milligrams

Potassium: 3,500 milligrams

Protein: 50 grams

Eating right

the well-known secret to good health

There are simple, basic guidelines for maintaining a balanced diet that will help you feel better and help you manage your IBS. They may not be new, but you have never before had a more compelling reason to follow them.

Eat a variety of foods. A healthy diet includes choices from each of the five different food groups: bread and cereals, fruits, vegetables, dairy products, and meats. Even if you find you have to cut out one type of food, such as wheat, it's still important to eat a variety of foods. If you find you can't drink milk, for instance, don't assume all dairy is out of range. Many people with lactose intolerance find they can still eat yogurt. Also, hard cheeses have less lactose than soft cheese and are usually easier to digest for those with lactose intolerance.

Cut down on fat and cholesterol. You already know that you need to cut down on fat, because it's often an IBS trigger. The American Heart Association recommends that people limit their fat intake to 30 percent of their daily calories. If you eat about 2,000 calories a day, that means 67 grams or less of fat daily and 200 milligrams of cholesterol a day.

Eat vegetables, fruits, and whole grains. They supply the carbohydrates that are the basic energy source for our bodies. Carbohydrates in general should make up 55 to 60 percent of your calories. But not all carbohydrates are created equal. Simple carbohydrates, such as refined sugar and honey, have few other nutrients. You'll get a quick (but short-lived) energy boost from a candy bar, but not much else (except maybe a bout of diarrhea or stomach cramps from the sorbitol or fructose sugars). You digest it quickly, which drives up your blood sugar but strains your insulin-producing pancreas. Complex carbohydrates, on the other hand—fruits, vegetables, and whole grain products, like high-fiber bread—are digested more slowly, are lower in fat, and create a sensation of fullness. If you eat a piece of whole wheat bread, for example, you'll get energy, but also vitamins, minerals, fiber, and some protein. And fiber is very important for minimizing IBS symptoms.

Keep sugar and salt to a minimum. You already know that there are certain sugars you probably should avoid. But sodium, or salt, can also be a no-no. Sodium causes your body to retain water, making you feel bloated and uncomfortable. It can also negatively affect your blood pressure. Yet most Americans get more than three teaspoons (8,000 milligrams, or 8 grams) of salt each day. Most comes not from salt shakers, but from processed foods. That's why checking food labels is so important. If you see the words "salt," "soda," or "sodium" high up on the ingredient list, then the product contains high amounts of sodium. Dietitians, the U.S. Department of Health and Human Services, and the American Heart Association all recommend limiting your daily salt intake to half a teaspoon (2,400 milligrams).

Watch Your Portions

Proper serving size is very important to healthy eating. Many of us eat portions that are too big and supply too many calories. Portion sizes of packaged, take-out, and restaurant foods are simply too large and filled with too many calories. The solution is to cut back. Here is an easy guide to help you better estimate portion sizes:

1 serving of fruit: baseball

1 serving of cheese: 2 dominos

1 serving of meat, chicken: palm of a woman's hand

1 serving of vegetables/starches: bulb part of a light bulb

Exercise and IBS

how moving your body helps with IBS

For many people with IBS, getting just a little bit of exercise seems impossible. This is understandable. It's hard to feel like exercising when you have stomach cramps or have to spend most mornings in the bathroom. All you want to do is lie down and hope this all goes away. Alas, the problem with any chronic disorder is that it rarely just goes away on its own. You need to take action. One of the best things you can do is try a bit of exercise. When you exercise, your body releases endorphins—hormones that make you feel good all over—and, as a result, your stress level shrinks. More to the point, if you have constipation-predominant IBS, exercise can help keep you regular. That's because exercise stimulates bowel activity, especially if done early in the morning when the bowel is at its most sluggish.

How to get started? Try fitness walking. It turns out to be the easiest and safest way to start. Just get a good pair of walking shoes and walk out the door. Better yet, call a friend and take a walk together. If you're a new fitness walker, start with a 10-minute walk. After a month or so, add two or three minutes until you can walk for a full 30 minutes. How fast should you walk? Start out slowly, and gradually work up to a 12- to 15-minute mile. You'll burn off twice as many calories at that pace as you would walking a 20-minute mile. To walk the walk, take short strides so you don't have to push off too hard with your back foot. Lean forward slightly from your ankles when you're walking at an easy or moderate pace; when you pick up the pace, lean forward from your hips. If being away from the facilities worries you, consider getting a treadmill.

If you have difficulty walking, then consider swimming. It's a great aerobic activity because your buoyancy in water takes the strain off your body. You can get great strength training and cardio workouts with little impact. If you choose to swim one or two times a week in a pool, take extra care of your skin and hair to offset sensitivities from the chlorine.

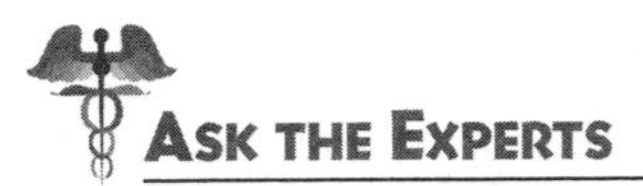

Ask the Experts

I always start a fitness program with the best of intentions, but then in a few weeks' time I am back to my old frumpy ways of no exercise. How can I make myself stick with it?

The number one reason most people give up on their exercise program is lack of time. To combat that easy out, incorporate your fitness into life and not against it. In other words, you want to make your fitness routine the equivalent of brushing your teeth at night—a steady habit that feels awkward to go without. Start by walking around your house or the parking lot at work for at least five to ten minutes before work, then again at lunchtime, and yet again in the early evening or right after work. The second reason people quit is boredom. Enlist a partner in your fitness program and make it fun.

I have never worked out before. Should I see my doctor first?

That depends on your health status. If you have never exercised before and, in addition to your IBS, have a health condition (for example, high blood pressure or joint problems or a previous injury), it is a good idea to check with your doctor before you sign up for a workout regime. Chances are, however, your doctor has been urging you to "get active" and will applaud your efforts. Just start out slowly and go at your own pace.

Helpful resources

American Dietetic Association Complete Food and Nutrition Guide
by Roberta Larson Duyff, M.S., R.D., C.F.C.S.
Sound advice on eating, including chapters on nutrition and health conditions and dietary supplements

Tell Me What to Eat If I Have Irritable Bowel Syndrome
by Elaine Magee, M.P.H., R.D.
Filled with good advice and recipes

American Dietetic Association
800-877-1600
www.eatright.org
Offers nutrition information, including consumer tips, fact sheets, FAQs, resources, and referrals for dietitians.

Chapter 7

Women and IBS

IBS and menstruation 118

Zelnorm and Lotronex 120

Pain and women 122

Pregnancy and IBS 124

IBS in women vs. men 126

Helpful resources 128

IBS and menstruation

charting symptoms by your cycle

For many women, the menstrual cycle comes with a host of menstrual-related symptoms—from painful abdominal cramps to bloating. If the discomfort is severe enough, doctors consider it a disorder known as **pre-menstrual syndrome**. It is due to the sudden drop-off of the reproductive hormones, estrogen and progesterone, right before menstruation. This hormonal free fall can play havoc with your moods, your digestion, your sleep patterns, and your pain threshold. Small wonder women with PMS report feeling out of commission for a few days before and during their period. Researchers surmise that the plummeting levels of hormones also play a role in IBS. How else to explain the fact that one-half to three-fourths of women with IBS say their symptoms get worse during their periods? And studies have proven them right: women with IBS have worse abdominal pain and bloating during menstruation than during other parts of their cycle. They also have more frequent bowel movements. Plus, women get the feeling they're going to have a bowel movement, called **rectal sensitivity**, more often and stronger during menstruation than during other phases of their cycle.

There's also some thinking that **prostaglandin**, a hormonelike substance the uterus makes during menstruation, may have something to do with the increase in IBS symptoms. Prostaglandins affect smooth muscle and are responsible for the cramps many women experience during their periods. Prostaglandins also line the intestinal walls; thus menstruation may sensitize the intestines as well.

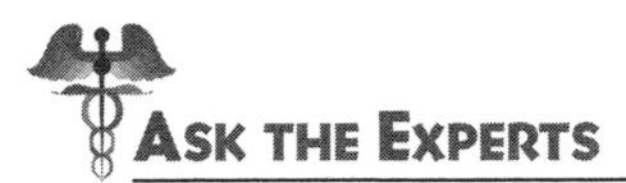

Ask the Experts

Can I expect my IBS symptoms to improve once I go through menopause?

Although the overall incidence of gastrointestinal problems, such as colon cancer, diverticulosis, and pelvic floor dysfunction, increases after menopause, there's no evidence that IBS symptoms get worse. They may even improve, thanks to sharply reduced levels of estrogen and progesterone. One study of more than 800 patients found that the increased severity of symptoms that women experience compared to men fades, with postmenopausal women reporting the same level of symptoms as men. Some studies even find that IBS in women becomes less common after menopause.

My doctor suggested birth control pills to help regulate my menstruation-related IBS symptoms. I've had my tubes tied, so I can't get pregnant. Why would I need to be on birth control pills?

Oral contraceptives are a synthetic form of your body's own hormones, organized in such a way as to prevent you from ovulating, or releasing an egg. This, in turn, prevents the corresponding peaks in progesterone and estrogen that can make your IBS symptoms worse. Women whose periods are irregular or very heavy or very light, or who experience strong cramps, are often put on oral contraceptives to regulate their cycles. You may find you have less pain and fewer symptoms while taking birth control pills. If your doctor is recommending it, it might be worth a try!

Zelnorm and Lotronex

women-only drugs for now

Very few drugs discriminate on the basis of gender, but that's the case with the two FDA-approved medications for the treatment of IBS in women: Zelnorm and Lotronex. Neither is approved for use in men. Why? In studies including men, the drugs didn't appear to work as well in men as in women. Both drugs zero in on **serotonin**, a neurotransmitter, or chemical messenger, in the brain and gut. New research shows that some 95 percent of serotonin is actually found in the gut. And that too little serotonin can contribute to constipation, while too much can cause diarrhea. To that end, drug researchers have worked to find ways to use serotonin to treat various types of IBS.

In women whose main IBS complaint is constipation, researchers have found that one particular serotonin-4 receptor can help by activating serotonin in the gut. Marketed under the brand name Zelnorm, this serotonin-4 receptor works to normalize colonic transit time and reduce abdominal pain.

Women with severe diarrhea-predominant IBS now have recourse to a drug called Lotronex. It works by blocking one type of serotonin receptor (the 5-HT3 receptor), which brings a halt to diarrhea and pain. This drug, however, can have a rare but life-threatening side effect: ischemic colitis. If there is rectal pain or sudden worsening of abdominal pain, see your doctor immediately.

So, will the drugs work in men? In the few trials that did have enough men to come up with a statistically significant figure, the answer is yes. But both drugs have the potential for significant, possibly dangerous, side effects. Given the lack of evidence on the effects on men, the FDA decided to restrict their use to women, where the results were clearer. Eventually, however, as more studies are conducted in men with IBS, that may change.

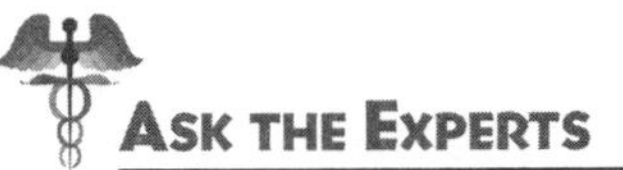

Ask the Experts

My old doctor prescribed Lotronex for my diarrhea-predominant IBS. It worked wonders, but he has retired and I can't find another doctor to prescribe it. What can I do?

Lotronex has a checkered history. It was approved in early 2000 by the FDA and then pulled off the market eight months later after reports of at least four deaths and nearly 200 serious cases of ischemic colitis, a dangerous condition where there is a decreased blood flow to the intestines. But for many women, it was the only medicine that helped solve their chronic IBS diarrhea. Strong patient advocacy brought the drug back onto the market in 2002, the first time ever that a drug already withdrawn was allowed to be sold again. However, the FDA put significant restrictions on its use, such as requiring that patients and their doctors complete special forms before filling a prescription. Many doctors are loath to prescribe Lotronex lest, even with these written safeguards, their patients experience problems. Call your local hospital and ask to speak to the gastroenterologist on staff. He or she may be able to offer a referral.

Pain and women

why women hurt more

Researchers have found that a woman's hormone levels influence her pain tolerance. When estrogen levels are highest—just before menstruation and during pregnancy and labor—women's brains are better at activating internal "antipain" mechanisms, including the release of extra "feel good" endorphins. The lower a woman's estrogen levels, the more sensitive she may be to menstrual and labor pain, as well as painful stimuli from the gastrointestinal system. This adds fuel to the theory that women may process the pain of IBS differently than men.

Studies also find that men and women respond differently to pain relievers. In one study conducted at the University of California at San Francisco, for instance, researchers found that women who received morphinelike painkillers called kappa opioids after having their wisdom teeth removed reported more powerful and long-lasting pain relief than men.

Sexual Intercourse and IBS

Sex can often be painful for women with IBS, possibly due to their increased pain perception and possibly to other aspects of the disease, such as fatigue, bloating, and constipation. Also, women with IBS may be embarrassed to have sex, worried that they'll have an accident or release gas during intercourse. In a British study, 45 percent of IBS sufferers surveyed said IBS negatively affected their sex lives.

But having IBS shouldn't mean a life without sex. Here is some hard-won advice on how to stay sexually active:

- **Time your lovemaking.** If you can, plan your lovemaking. Choose a time before you've eaten or several hours after a meal. This should reduce the risk of flatulence or other embarrassing sounds, and reduce the likelihood of any sudden need for the bathroom.

- **Use humor.** After all, all women, at some point, make embarrassing sounds during sex. Turn any incidents into a joke and you will relieve much of your embarrassment.

- **Be honest with your partner.** Tell him or her about your condition and what might happen during sex.

- **Find other ways to be intimate.** Sex isn't always the answer. How about a stress-relieving massage with a scented oil? A bubble bath with your partner?

Pregnancy and IBS

how hormones during pregnancy affect IBS

IBS does not necessarily abate with pregnancy. In most cases, it follows a woman into her pregnancy—and may make the normal discomfort of pregnancy even worse. That's because during pregnancy the levels of various hormones that can directly affect your digestion are raised. The increased levels of progesterone and estrogen during pregnancy slow things down in the digestive system. Plus, relaxin, a hormone released by the placenta to quiet smooth-muscle contractions and prevent premature labor, affects the smooth muscle in the digestive system, as well. The result is usually constipation for most women, especially in their last trimester.

Pregnancy can exacerbate any kind of IBS, be it predominant constipation or diarrhea. (In fact, pregnancy has been known to cause gas, bloating, and other IBS symptoms in many women who do not have IBS.) Because good nutrition is vital at this time for both your health and your baby's health, you need to be especially vigilant about what you eat. You need to have a well-rounded diet that is high in calcium and fiber. If you have diarrhea-predominant IBS, you may find that pregnancy will offer some relief.

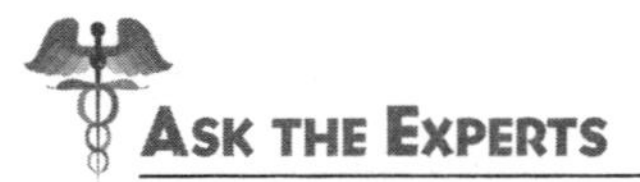

Ask the Experts

Are any of the drugs currently used for IBS safe for use during pregnancy?

Few drugs are ever specifically tested for safety in pregnant women because such research would be considered unethical. Instead, what doctors know about medication use during pregnancy comes from women who have voluntarily used the drugs during their pregnancy. Within the family of drugs used for IBS, anticholinergics, Zelnorm, and Lotronex have proven safe in animal studies. This doesn't mean you should continue taking them if you are pregnant, or thinking about getting pregnant, without first talking to your doctor.

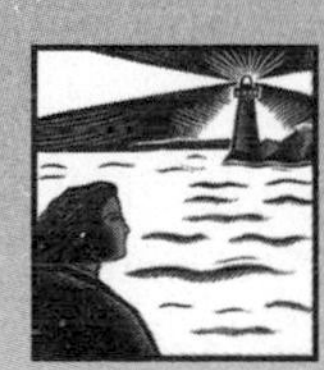

FIRST PERSON INSIGHTS

IBS-free pregnancies

During my pregnancies, I had only a few bouts of IBS diarrhea in the first trimester. After that, my IBS seemed to go into remission and I remained symptom-free for another year after each baby was born. But each time, my IBS returned, worse than ever. I always wondered was it the stress of caring for young children? During my pregnancies, particularly early on with the diarrhea, I made sure to drink plenty of water so I didn't become dehydrated. I also cut my work hours back to part-time so I could get extra rest and not become overly stressed. Once each of my kids turned one, I returned to work and my IBS got worse. I now wonder if the pregnancy-imposed stress-reduction is what helped with the IBS.

Serena F., Iowa City, IA

IBS in women vs. men

why 70 percent of those with IBS are women

Given the fact that women in the United States are twice as likely as men to be diagnosed with IBS, you could draw the logical conclusion that this condition is found mainly in women, much like fibromyalgia or chronic fatigue syndrome. While this is indeed true, the extreme discrepancy in the diagnosis of IBS in men and women may also be because American women are more likely than men to visit a health care professional about IBS symptoms.

Two other strong correlations between women and IBS show that it is indeed primarily a woman's disorder. The first is that estrogen and progesterone are clearly involved in IBS. Researchers are investigating just how these hormones influence the digestive process.

Second, there is a very strong correlation between IBS and sexual and/or physical abuse in childhood. Up to 50 percent of women with severe IBS were abused as children. These women also often have **posttraumatic stress disorder**. The symptoms of this disorder vary, but nearly always involve some form of depression. (In cases of clinical depression, medical treatment should always be sought.)

Researchers think that the trauma of being abused as a child (for men or women) may trigger powerful long-lasting disturbances in the gut that can lead to IBS and, in many cases, depression as well. In such cases, antidepressants may be especially helpful. See pages 72–73 for more on the brain/gut connection.

IBS in Women

◆ Women are just as likely as men to suffer from any of the three subtypes of IBS: with diarrhea, with constipation, or pain predominant.

◆ Symptoms of IBS typically occur in women between ages 30 and 50, with an average age of 29.

◆ Women with IBS have a greater risk of unnecessary surgery, particularly hysterectomy or ovarian surgery, than women without the condition.

◆ Women with IBS experience symptoms an average of 194 days a year, or about 16 days a month. About 25 percent experience symptoms every single day.

◆ Two-thirds of women report "bathroom anxiety," always needing to know where the closest bathroom is.

◆ Women with IBS seem to have more bloating, nausea, and constipation, whereas men with IBS report more diarrhea.

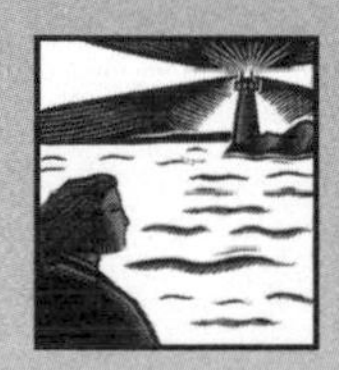

FIRST PERSON INSIGHTS

It's not IBS

I had bloating, intense abdominal pain and cramps, and diarrhea. I thought it was food poisoning and so did my doctor. He sent me to a gastroenterologist, who ran a battery of tests and concluded that I probably had irritable bowel syndrome, except that I was in my late 40s and IBS doesn't usually start then. Also, I had an enlarged abdomen, which made me look like I was five months pregnant. Unlike most IBS symptoms, which wax and wane, my belly was always enlarged. My doctor ordered more tests. An X-ray of my abdomen revealed nothing, but a CAT scan showed fluid in my abdomen, which is not normal. My doctor took a sample of this fluid and found cancer cells. Then he ran a CA 125 blood test, and I was diagnosed with ovarian cancer. Because it was found early, the cancer had not spread and I have a great chance for a full recovery. I am so glad my doctor persisted in finding the right diagnosis.

Mary K., San Diego, CA

Helpful resources

Digestive Wellness
by Elizabeth Lipski, M.S., C.C.N.

The Irritable Bowel Syndrome (IBS) & Gastrointestinal Solutions Handbook
by Chet Cunningham

What You Really Need to Know About Irritable Bowel Syndrome
by Robert Buckman, M.D., and Nigel Howard (editor)

IBS Health
www.ibshealth.com

Whole HealthMD
www.wholehealthmd.com/hc/resourceareas_view/1,1438,484,00.html

National Library of Medicine: IBS
www.nlm.nih.gov/medlineplus/irritablebowelsyndrome.html
Easy-to-read articles on IBS diagnosis, treatment, and other related issues.

Chapter 8

Children and IBS

What the doctor needs to know 130

Diagnosing IBS 132

A personal treatment plan 134

Stress in children 136

Helpful resources 138

What the doctor needs to know
and what parents can do to help

As every parent knows, stomach aches are common in children. All sorts of things can cause them, be it one too many hot dogs or a spelling test. In most cases, the tummy trouble passes and your child is soon back to normal. But what if those tummy aches continue to occur on a regular basis? Then it is time to seek medical help. Childhood stomach pain—just like adult stomach pain—deserves a thorough medical evaluation. Here is what typically will happen.

Your child's pediatrician should first take a careful medical history. This involves asking you and your child (depending on his or her age) questions about his or her stomach pain and bathroom habits. The doctor may ask questions about past illnesses or injuries, when the child first began experiencing stomach problems, and what the stomach problems have been like since. Common questions include

- Where is the pain located?
- Any vomiting associated with the pain?
- Does the pain wake your child up at night?

The doctor will probably also ask you numerous questions about your child's recent stomach aches and what has been going on in your child's life.

- What is going on at school? Is your child getting a lot of homework, having trouble with tests, having problems with a teacher?
- What is going on with friends? Is your child fighting with friends, being teased, having problems with bullying?
- Does exercise or playing make the stomach ache worse?
- What does your child do when he or she has a stomach ache?

Don't be surprised if the doctor asks you to leave the room while she talks to your child. Because psychological stress can play such a major role in functional disorders like IBS, the doctor may want to ask the child some questions that might be easier for him or her to answer with you out of the room. This is particularly true of adolescents. It's also important that the doctor hear your child describe the symptoms in his or her own words. Too often, parents have a tendency to answer for their children.

Recurrent Abdominal Pain

Between 10 and 25 percent of school-age children and adolescents experience a condition called **recurrent abdominal pain**, or RAP. It is the most common functional bowel disorder seen in children. RAP is defined as three or more episodes of abdominal pain severe enough to interfere with a child's regular activities during a three-month period. This differs from IBS because problems with bowel movements (diarrhea or constipation) are not required for the doctor to reach a diagnosis. Researchers suspect that about 90 percent of RAP in children is related to psychosomatic causes.

Yet a significant number of children with RAP also meet the criteria for IBS. In fact, one study of 225 children with RAP found that 68 percent met the criteria used in adults to diagnose IBS. Additionally, long-term studies find that symptoms of RAP persist into adulthood, and that adults with IBS often have a history of childhood abdominal pain.

Diagnosing IBS

never too young to have it

As with adults, there is no clinical test to determine if your child has IBS. Some doctors consider it a diagnosis of exclusion in children. If they can't find anything else that's organically wrong, they diagnose the child with IBS. Still, it's important that your doctor conduct the necessary tests to rule out other conditions that share many symptoms with IBS, such as inflammatory bowel disease, infection, lactose intolerance, and celiac disease. These are described in more detail on pages 12–15. Each requires specific evaluations to reach a diagnosis, including blood tests and X-rays. Whether or not your doctor conducts these tests depends on your child's actual symptoms. No doctor wants to put a child through unnecessary tests.

If your child has no fever, weight loss, vomiting, blood in the stool, or poor growth, doctors usually diagnosis IBS and treat the child for the disorder. If, however, the child continues to have significant problems even with IBS treatment, the doctor may conduct additional tests.

A diagnosis of IBS in children is based on abdominal pain or discomfort plus any two of the following:

- The pain is relieved with a bowel movement.
- The beginning of the pain correlates with a change in stool frequency.
- The beginning of the pain correlates with a change in the consistency of the stool (either harder or softer).

These symptoms must be present for at least 12 weeks over the past year, with no disease or other physical changes causing the symptoms.

Unlike IBS in adults, which affects twice as many women as men, IBS in children appears to affect boys and girls equally. Each is just as likely to have diarrhea-predominant or constipation-predominant IBS, or to have a variable stool pattern (both diarrhea and constipation).

Children with IBS may also have headaches or nausea, or have mucus in their stool. One study found weekly headaches in more than half of adolescents with frequent abdominal pain, but in just one-fourth of those without it. A similar study conducted in Sweden on children from first through ninth grades found the same results.

Children with IBS may also lose weight because they often refuse to eat, fearing that eating will cause their stomach problems to get worse.

As with adults, symptoms in children can come after a significant stressful event, such as teething or problems at home, or an infectious disease, such as the flu. Also, as with adults, while stress can make IBS in children worse, it doesn't cause it.

A personal treatment plan

tailor medication and lifestyle changes to a child's life

Before beginning any treatment, you and your child's doctor will first clarify the intensity and pattern of your child's irritable bowel syndrome. Is it diarrhea predominant? Constipation predominant? Predominantly painful? Does it tend to get worse on school days or at night? This is where the symptom diary will come in handy.

The three keys in treating children, says pediatric gastroenterologist Jeffrey Hyams, M.D., who heads the Division of Digestive Diseases and Nutrition at Connecticut Children's Medical Center in Hartford, are diet, reassurance, and medication. Getting adequate dietary fiber is the first step, he says, particularly for those with constipation-predominant symptoms.

How much fiber? This depends on the age of the child. For children older than 3, add enough dietary fiber to equal their age plus 5. So a 4-year-old should have nine grams of fiber daily; a 10-year-old should have 15 grams. Good sources of fiber for children are whole fruits (try cutting them up so kids can nosh on them like candy), whole wheat products like bread and pasta (ditch the white bread), and snack foods like popcorn.

If your child has diarrhea-predominant IBS, avoid foods that contain the sugar sorbitol, such as certain juices and candies, and foods with high fructose corn syrup (even fast food hamburger buns are made with corn syrup). These two sweeteners are found in some unexpected places, including many juices, ketchup, and all sweets (except naturally sweet foods like dried and fresh fruits). Be sure to read food labels carefully.

Also avoid caffeine. You might think this would be easy with children, but caffeine can also turn up in some unexpected places, like certain granola snack bars and cereals, as well as sodas.

Depending on the severity of your child's symptoms, your doctor may decide to prescribe medication. The most commonly used medications in children are antispasmodics, such as dicyclomine or hyoscyamine, which work by relaxing the intestinal muscle. For older children with more severe symptoms, low doses of an antidepressant such as Elavil (amitriptyline) can help relieve pain. For more on the role of antidepressants and IBS, see pages 72–73.

Finally, counseling is critical, particularly when it is clear that events occurring in the child's life affect his or her IBS. For instance, if you and your spouse are going through a divorce or moving, or someone in the family is ill or has lost a job, your child's IBS may get worse, even if she keeps insisting that "nothing is bothering me!"

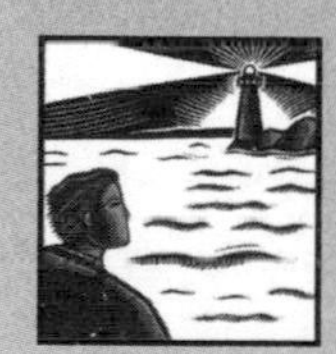

FIRST PERSON INSIGHTS

Coping at school

I have IBS and so does a really close friend of mine. Sometimes we talk about how we are doing, though he doesn't like to talk about it that much. Probably because at the high school he goes to, he gets teased about having to go to the bathroom all the time. So he hates school. He won't even let his mother tell his teacher about it. But I decided that I wasn't going to keep my IBS a secret. I told two of my teachers about my IBS. It took a lot of courage, but they were great about it.

If I don't feel well, one teacher lets me go to the nurse so I can lie down for a while, or to the library where it's quiet and I can work without getting uptight, which always makes my IBS worse. Sometimes I don't feel well enough to go to school, but my teachers are very good about sending work home, or even e-mailing my assignments so I don't fall too far behind. So long as I show that I am doing my work and trying, they are on my side. I think the key is being really honest about what is happening with you.

Jeremy K., age 14, Atlanta, GA

Stress in children
often hidden, yet always there

Although, as you know, stress doesn't cause IBS, it definitely plays a role in its exacerbation, triggering IBS episodes and pain. This is particularly true with children who often lead overscheduled, overcommitted lives, racing from piano lessons to soccer practices to after-school tutoring. They are under tremendous pressure to succeed in and out of school and often have very little downtime to just be kids. Even watching television and playing video games, with their high levels of violence and mature topics, can inadvertently add to a child's stress levels.

If your child has IBS, these high levels of stress can be devastating. It is important that you work to reduce the amount of stress and activity in your child's life and also teach your child how to better handle stress. One study found that children with chronic abdominal pain (such as the kind of pain that comes with IBS) can be helped with **guided imagery therapy**. Guided imagery therapy combines relaxation, imagery, and hypnosis to help children gain control of their pain. (For more on complementary therapies, see Chapter 11.) It works by affecting the autonomic nervous system—the same nerves that play a role in the digestive system and significantly contribute to IBS.

Don't underestimate the stress that IBS itself will cause your child. Children are often very embarrassed about the symptoms, an embarrassment they may go out of their way to hide from you as well as their friends. Keeping the condition secret and feeling shame about it creates its own stress. So encourage your child to talk about her condition and to share her concerns with you while at the same time respecting her privacy.

STEP BY STEP

Helping Your Child Cope with Stress

1. Make a list of all the activities your child is doing and the expectations you hold for your child. Find places to cut out scheduled activities to provide your child with more downtime.

2. Examine your own schedule. Are you working excessively? Taking on too many volunteer activities? Children pick up on your stress and take it on themselves.

3. Find 10 minutes a day (at least) to spend with your child—just the two of you. Play a quiet game together, or read aloud to your child. It is often during these quiet one-on-one times that children open up to their parents and tell them what is really going on.

4. Provide consistency and routines for your child.

5. Make sure your child is getting enough exercise and is following a nutritious diet that does not exacerbate her IBS.

6. Help your child recognize when she is feeling stressed. Work together to find a routine that helps abate the stress. You might want to consider teaching your child how to practice deep breathing (see pages 178–179) or other stress-reducing techniques.

7. Take a good hard look at your own behavior toward your child. Are you overly demanding, critical, or controlling?

Helpful resources

Your Digestive System (How Your Body Works)
by Anita Ganeri

Stomachaches (My Health)
by Alvin Silverstein, et al.

Eating and Digestion (Body Systems)
by Angela Royston

The First Year—IBS (Irritable Bowel Syndrome): An Essential Guide for the Newly Diagnosed
by Heather Van Vorous

www.aap.org
The American Academy of Pediatrics provides pertinent information on a variety of health topics of interest to parents, from digestive problems and nutrition to safety tips.

About Kids GI Disorders
www.aboutkidsgi.org

CHAPTER 9

Using the Internet

Evaluating Web sites 140

Top IBS health sites for consumers 142

Top medical sites on IBS 144

Researching doctors 146

Alternative approaches 148

Online support 150

Newsgroups 152

Helpful resources 154

Evaluating Web sites

sorting the good from the bad

The Internet is an amazing resource. So it's only natural that once you receive a diagnosis of irritable bowel syndrome you head to your computer and log on, searching for any and all information you can find. That's a good instinct—hold on to it.

But before you go into cyberspace, you need to become an informed consumer of Internet health sites. Why? Because not every health site is created equal. Some sites may contain outdated facts, misinformation, poor research, urban legends, propaganda, and outright lies.

So how can you tell what's good and what's not? Use this checklist.

✔ **Check the date.** In a book or newspaper, you can always see the publication date, so you know whether the information is current. On the Web, not every page carries the publication date. The better medical sites do. If you don't see a date, don't trust any figures the page calls "current." Sometimes the date of an article can be found in its Web address.

✔ **Check the source.** Most articles online have bylines giving the writer's name. If you have not heard of the writer, feed the name into a search engine and see what other sites carry the byline. A good medical paper always backs up its statements with sources and bibliographies. Check any article for sources and links to other sites.

✔ **Check the publisher.** Look at the Web address of any article you are evaluating. Is it a name you recognize—a well-known clinic or foundation or government site? If not, look around for a link labeled "About this site," or something similar, and see who is behind it.

✔ **Don't be put off by advertising.** Advertising is a fact of life on the Web. One exception: If a site seems to be selling something in its articles, move on. You cannot trust advertorials on television, so don't trust your health to them online.

Print Out Only What You Need

Great. You just hit a page with handy links and lots of good solid information. Instead of stopping to write down the name of the site, you have several options for saving the information:

Bookmark the page. Every Web browser lets you save the names of favorite Web pages. In Internet Explorer, click on Favorites; in America Online, click on Favorite Places; and in Netscape, click on Bookmarks. Next time you want to access that page, all you need to do is look through your list of favorite sites or bookmarks and click on it.

Print the page. When you find a page with relevant information, print it out and file it in your health journal (see pages 24–25). As the number of printouts grows, you can categorize them by topic: medicine, specialists, alternative therapies, diet, and so on. This will make it easier to find the information. Remember: You don't have to print an entire Web page. Just highlight the bit that interests you, click on File, then Print, and in the Print box, click on Selection. Then click on the OK button or "Apply" and you'll have a nice short printout.

File the page. You can save copies of Web pages to your hard drive. Just click on the File tab in the toolbar, then "Save as," and then direct the computer to save it in whichever folder you want. You can set up a folder called IBS, and then create subfolders with a specific focus, such as diet, stress reduction, and alternative therapies.

Top IBS health sites for consumers

the best sites to start with

With millions of Web sites, many of them devoted to health information, searching the Internet can quickly become overwhelming. As someone coping with an already overwhelming health condition, more stress is the last thing you need. So start with these well-known IBS sites, considered to be the best on the Web.

www.iffgd.org

The International Foundation for Functional Gastrointestinal Disorders is a nonprofit organization designed to provide education and support services to pediatricians, family practitioners, specialists, nurses, home health care companies, and most importantly, children and families living with GI disorders. It also supports ongoing research into functional gastrointestinal disorders.

www.aboutibs.org

Start here for information and support about IBS and you may not even need another site. About IBS, sponsored by the International Foundation for Functional Gastrointestinal Disorders, contains information about the diagnosis, treatment, and prognosis of IBS, bulletin boards for support and online chatting, special online guests who can answer your questions in real time, and a plethora of facts and tips about living with IBS that should make any IBS patient's life easier.

www.aboutkidsgi.org

This Web site is also run and sponsored by the International Foundation for Functional Gastrointestinal Disorders, with a specific focus on GI disorders like IBS in children. Browse it for research updates and helpful advice; with an individual or family member subscription, you can receive informative publications.

www.gastro.org

The American Gastroenterological Association is a professional society that provides training and educational support for gastroenterologists. But the AGS Web site also has special sections for patients, providing valuable information about various digestive diseases, including IBS, as well as press releases and summaries of some of the latest research.

www.ibsassociation.org

A nonprofit organization dedicated to helping those who suffer from IBS through patient support groups, treatment, accurate information and education, the Irritable Bowel Syndrome Association offers updates on medical research, treatments, new books about IBS, and clinical studies on IBS.

Smart searching tips

Make every search count. It's important to use precise search terms, or keywords. The more words you type in, the more specific your search will be. Entering more keywords increases the relevance of what you get in return, but also limits the number of returns you'll see. Try a broad search first, then narrow down the results by adding search terms.

Each search engine typically has a link that takes you to an "advanced" search form. There, you can refine your search by entering words you don't want to see—for instance, excluding the word "depressed" if you want to read only about the physical aspects of IBS.

Put quotes around words that should appear next to each other, and the search engine will treat them as one word. Searching for "disability insurance" will help you find pages that refer to that specific type of insurance, rather than pages that cover insurance in general and disabilities in general.

Top medical sites on IBS

go to these for clinical information

Once you have a basic grounding in IBS, you'll be ready to sink your teeth into some more detailed information. Instead of wasting time with general searches, go to one of the following medical sites for in-depth information on IBS, treatments, research, and clinical trials. These sites—maintained by major medical institutions or the U.S. government—provide some of the best and most trustworthy information available online.

Medline Plus

www.nlm.nih.gov/medlineplus/irritablebowelsyndrome.html

This government Web site offers an excellent starting point for government and other reputable information about IBS.

National Institute of Diabetes & Digestive & Kidney Diseases

www.niddk.nih.gov

This government agency conducts and supports research on many of the most serious diseases affecting public health. The site includes patient information on a variety of digestive diseases, including IBS.

American Academy of Family Physicians

www.aafp.org, or the slightly more user-friendly **www.familydoctor.org**

Both sites are sponsored by the same organization, and both offer solid information for patients as well as sections for professionals. The sites include reader-friendly definitions and articles spanning everything from the best nutritional program to an overview of treatment options.

Journal of the American Medical Association (JAMA)

www.jama.ama-assn.org

The Web site for this esteemed publication is updated daily and contains excellent abstracts on various aspects of IBS.

Mayo Clinic

www.mayoclinic.com

The subtitle says it all: "reliable information for a healthier life." This easy-to-navigate site from a well-respected institute offers comprehensive information not only on IBS and related syndromes but on virtually any health issue, from living with chronic pain to finding the right doctor, as well as explanations on complementary and alternative medicines.

The American College of Gastroenterology

www.acg.gi.org

With sections geared for both patients and medical professionals, this site offers solid explanations and definitions on IBS, as well as a national directory of gastroenterologists.

Intelihealth

www.intelihealth.com

Operated in conjunction with Harvard Medical School, with all content screened by Harvard experts (and, in many cases, written by them), this is an excellent site for information on a variety of health conditions.

National Women's Health Resource Center

www.healthywomen.org

Geared toward women, this exceptionally reader-friendly site, owned and operated by the nonprofit organization, contains explanations for just about any condition, disease, or syndrome you can name, including IBS. All content is verified and vetted by some of the top medical experts in the field.

Go Ask Alice!

www.goaskalice.columbia.edu

This is Columbia University's question and answer site. Supported by a team of Columbia University health educators and health care providers, along with information and research specialists from health-related organizations worldwide, it archives previous questions so you can read earlier posts. The site has its own search engine and receives more than 1,500 questions a week on every conceivable health topic. Do a search on "irritable bowel syndrome" for numerous answers to questions you may have.

Researching doctors

where to find the right medical help

For many years, IBS was considered a purely psychological condition. Unfortunately, too many doctors still adhere to that kind of outdated thinking. So finding the right doctor, one who understands that your condition is not just stress related, is important. The Internet offers a terrific place to research and find the right doctor. While the Net can't reveal a doctor's bedside manner or level of compassion, it can turn up his or her educational background, professional credentials, publications, research, and any disciplinary actions against him.

The American Gastroenterological Association (AGA)

www.gastro.org

Most experts agree that gastroenterologists are among the best-trained specialists to deal with IBS. On this site, you can find a gastroenterologist within a specific state. Keep in mind, however, that all data in the AGA's database is self-reported, and the organization does not verify the accuracy, completeness, timeliness, or appropriateness of the information, nor does it endorse doctors listed there. That part is up to you, with the help of the following sites.

The American Medical Association (AMA)

www.ama-assn.org

You can search for information, including educational background, on a physician based upon medical specialty, name, or location.

American Board of Medical Specialties (ABMS)

www.abms.org

This is an organization of 24 medical specialty boards that will tell you whether a doctor is board certified or board eligible in a particular area. "Board certified" means a doctor has completed additional years of training and passed a national examination. "Board eligible" means the doctor has completed the training, but not the test.

Best Doctors

www.bestdoctors.com

This site charges a fee to search its database, but it verifies all the information about the physicians in its database and undertakes an annual review of all doctors to determine if they have been the subjects of disciplinary actions by state medical boards. If they have, they are usually deleted from the database. The site does not charge physicians who are in the database, and it finds the "best doctors" by asking other physicians whom they would see for a specific medical condition. The news program *60 Minutes* said, "Best Doctors is changing the face of American medicine." The site has about 30,000 physicians—about 4 percent of all doctors in the U.S.—in its database.

Pain Net, Inc.

www.painnet.com

Describing itself as the "JD Power, Nielsen Ratings, Consumer Reports of Pain," this organization advocates a comprehensive approach to pain management. It also offers a state-by-state listing of doctors, dentists, therapists, chiropractors, pharmacists, and counselors with training and education in treating painful diseases and conditions.

National Mental Health Association (NMHA)

www.nmha.org

This is the country's oldest and largest nonprofit organization addressing all aspects of mental health, with more than 340 affiliates nationwide. Its resource center provides referrals for local treatment centers and lists of mental health providers. It includes a toll-free hotline (800-969-6642).

Alternative approaches
looking outside the mainstream

If you're interested in learning more about various alternative therapies for IBS, your first stop should be organizations that take an out-of-the-mainstream approach to treatment of various diseases.

The Alternative Medicine Foundation

www.amfoundation.org

This site provides a primer on almost all forms of alternative treatment, including acupuncture, herbs, mind/body techniques, homeopathy, massage, and more. Much of the information contained on the site is free to the public, although there are some fee-based links.

American Holistic Health Organization

www.ahha.org

Feature articles, referral lists, and self-help information are the hallmarks of this site, which acts as a national clearinghouse for all things alternative. A great site to help you get associated with nontraditional approaches to care.

The National Center for Complementary and Alternative Medicine (NCCAM)

www.nccam.nih.gov

This government agency supports research on complementary and alternative medicine and helps demystify the alternatives by explaining which treatments work, which don't, and why. This site provides comprehensive information on alternative approaches integrated into traditional practices, as well as information on ongoing clinical trials of alternative approaches for a variety of conditions and diseases.

Note: You can find a significant amount of information on alternative treatments on IBS by typing "irritable bowel syndrome" and "alternative treatment" into any search engine. Be careful, however—much of the information is untested and may even be unsafe. A good source for information about dubious Web sites and treatments is Quack Watch, at **www.quackwatch.org**. This organization keeps tabs on fringe alternative treatments. And don't forget to talk to your primary doctor before trying anything you read about on the Internet.

Doctors and Internet-Savvy Patients

Much of the information you now have access to on the Internet was once the purview of doctors only. And until fairly recently, many doctors became frustrated with patients who arrived with armloads of studies and data about their condition. But today, most doctors have learned to appreciate a well-educated patient. Still, it's important that you present your information in the right manner, with the right attitude. Specifically:

◆ **Make it quick.** Time is money, and doctors don't have time to go through reams of data. If there's a study or treatment you're interested in, provide a quick summary, either verbally or in writing.

◆ **Provide your source.** Doctors know there's a lot of medical junk out there on the Internet. Make sure you provide information from a reputable source.

◆ **Don't be antagonistic.** Just because your doctor doesn't agree with your findings or hasn't heard about them before doesn't mean he or she is a bad doctor. Doctors are overwhelmed with information today, just like their patients.

◆ **Ask for help.** Many doctors today are Internet-savvy and can guide you to reputable sites.

Online support

welcome to the online world of IBS

When you learn that you have IBS, it can be a very lonely feeling. But in reality, one in five Americans has IBS—that's a lot of people experiencing the same kinds of issues you are. No surprise, they're looking for advice on what to eat, when to eat, how to cope with embarrassing symptoms, and what treatments work best. It's in this symptom sorting and solving that online support comes in handy.

Several Web sites offer online chat rooms where you can "talk" in virtual time to people who have IBS. At these sites, you'll find parents whose children have IBS, people your age with IBS, even people in your own area who might want to meet "in real life."

Just as with anything on the Internet, however, it's important to view the information you receive via these online groups with the proverbial grain of salt. If someone has a supplement she's trying to sell to cure IBS and she can tell you five studies have proved its efficacy and that it made a huge difference in her own life, beware. The age-old advice still holds: If it sounds too good to be true, it probably is.

If you find an online community you feel comfortable in, make sure to follow the rules set forth by that community. Some ask that you stick to the medical aspects of IBS only; others invite dialogue on anything you can imagine. Here are some good places to start.

www.ibsgroup.org

The largest and most active IBS self-help group, it formed in 1987 and its Web site launched in 1995. It is designed to support those who suffer from IBS, those looking for support for someone who has IBS, and medical professionals who want to learn more about IBS. The site gets more than 50,000 hits a month and offers support on topics ranging from diarrhea and constipation to diagnostic tests and adolescent issues.

iVillage

www.ivillage.com

Calling itself "the women's network—busy women sharing solutions and advice," this site has outstanding message boards and chat areas specifically geared toward those with IBS. It also contains easy-to-digest medical information, personal stories, and links to newsletters and articles.

Yahoo IBS group

groups.yahoo.com

Yahoo has several listserves devoted to IBS. Just type the words "irritable bowel syndrome" into the search box for a list. Joining is free. Some lists are moderated, meaning someone monitors the conversations to ensure they stay on topic and are conducted in a polite, appropriate manner; others are unmoderated, a kind of Wild West free-for-all. You can also search the archives of these lists once you sign up to see past "conversations."

Keeping Yourself Safe Online

When posting online, use a pseudonym and don't give your main e-mail address—it could open you up to lots of junk e-mail and spam. Instead, use a free account via Yahoo or Hotmail or Google specifically for these groups. Or, if you want to list your real e-mail address, spell out the @ sign as "at." This prevents programs called spiders that collect e-mails for junk mail from scooping up your address. Also, don't reveal too much personal information about yourself (address, phone number, real name) to someone you've just met online, even on a well-established IBS site. Take your time and go slowly, just as you would in any "real world" relationship.

Newsgroups

freewheeling give-and-take

In addition to online communities, there are newsgroups. These are essentially collections of e-mails, stored online for you to browse. You can post your own message by e-mailing it to the newsgroup. An easy way to access newsgroups is to click on Google's groups tab, then enter "irritable bowel syndrome." One newsgroup for IBS is **alt.support.ibs**.

Newsgroups, like Internet bulletin boards, are also a place to learn from others' mistakes, pick up advice, and post your own so others can benefit. As you start to scan the groups, you might notice that some responses to questions are met with derisive comments. Don't let Internet know-it-alls get you down. Take time to read the frequently asked questions (FAQs) available for most newsgroups so you don't ask a question that's been answered many times before. You can find FAQs for all newsgroups at **www.faqs.org**.

Ready to see if newsgroups are for you? All you need is an Internet connection and a Web browser, such as Internet Explorer, which is bundled free with every PC. Open your Web browser and type in alt.support.ibs. This should open a window in your e-mail program that will guide you through the setup process. You may need to check with your Internet provider to find out what address you need to type in for newsgroups. Most Internet providers provide this information on their home page. Remember: Don't use your real name and don't use your main e-mail address. You don't want to be inundated with spam or junk e-mail.

Once you've completed the setup process, in your e-mail program (Outlook, Eudora, AOL, etc.) you should see a section in your folders with the name of the newsgroup you just signed up for. Click on it and follow the directions for subscribing.

Once you fill in the registration form, follow the instructions. To post a message, click the "Post a new message" link on the main page, or when viewing someone else's message, click "Post a follow-up to this message." Then type in your message. If you want to see your message before sending it, click the "Preview message" button. Or click the "Post message no preview" button, if you're all set.

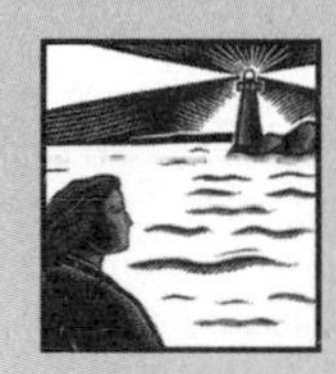

FIRST PERSON INSIGHTS

Virtual soulmates

Karen is one of my best friends, but I've never even met her in person! I don't even know what her voice sounds like. She and I met online in an IBS chat room. When I first received my diagnosis, I spent a lot of late nights online, looking for information on treatments, research—anything. I never expected to find a friend! At first, we talked a lot in a public chat area about IBS in general. But as we got to know and trust each other, we began exchanging personal e-mails.

Karen has helped me stay calm and take one day at a time. She's someone I can laugh with about the more "unique" moments of having IBS, and someone I can cry with when this disorder just seems more than I can bear. She understands how frustrating it is to try to live with a chronic illness like this and still try to be a mother to my three boys, take care of my husband, the house and the dog, and to work! She helps me see when I need to slow down and is quick to point out the connection between stress in my life and an IBS flare-up. I just don't know what I would have done if we hadn't met.

—Betsy S., Elmira, PA

Helpful resources

After Any Diagnosis: How to Take Action Against Your Illness Using the Best and Most Current Medical Information Available
by Carol Svec

The Health Resource
You don't have to search the Internet yourself. There are a number of companies that offer this service for a fee. One such company, called the Health Resource, does extensive Internet research compilation customized to your diagnosis. The company's Internet specialists comb through the Internet and other sources and locate medical articles geared toward your specific situation, including mainstream, experimental, and alternative treatments, along with top specialists. In a week to 10 days, you receive a hard copy of their booklet, complete with glossary. Prices range from $150 to $400.
800-949-0090
www.thehealthresource.com

Chapter 10

Stress and IBS

What is stress? 156

Chronic stress and IBS 158

Assault on mind and body 160

Smart IBS coping strategies 162

Take an IBS stress inventory 164

Learning to relax 166

Your partner's concerns 168

On the job 170

Helpful resources 172

What is stress?

it's not just a built-in survival mechanism

Stress has become the watchword for a number of medical problems today. In some cases, it is blamed for causing the health problem, for example, high blood pressure; in others, it is blamed for worsening symptoms. How can stress be both a cause and an effect? While scientists have learned a great deal about the nature of stress, what still puzzles them is that stress is in the eye of the beholder. In other words, how stress affects us is based mostly on how we perceive that stress. Some stressors help you perform at your peak ability; others can be debilitating. So far, the one thing researchers agree upon is that the primary reason for negative stress is the perception of not being in control. Not having control over one's life or environment can be a very threatening feeling, easily triggering the stress response.

A perceived short-term threat

This stressor could be a lunging tiger, an oncoming car, an angry boss, or an alarming physical symptom. Reacting to threats is so critical to your survival that your body is designed to either "fight or flee" the threat. Here's how it works: When you perceive a threat, a gland in your brain called the hypothalamus sends an alarm to your sympathetic nervous system to release adrenaline into your blood stream. At the same time, signals go out to speed up your heart rate and breathing, which provides you with the extra oxygen and blood supply you need to "fight or flee," but which also increases your blood pressure. While this response is intended to heighten your reaction to potentially dangerous situations, it doesn't bode well for rational thought or decision making. Also keep in mind that the perceived threat lies in the eye of the beholder. The stress response will occur whether the threat is real or imagined. (This is why your heart races during a scary movie.)

When you are under stress, your brain also signals the adrenal glands to release norepinephrine, another stress hormone. Together with adrenaline, also called epinephrine, this hormone increases glucose levels in your blood, sending extra energy to your cells so your muscles can respond better, and shutting down your digestive tract to conserve energy. This alert mechanism is what helps us survive a physical short-term threat; for example, running from an angry dog or swimming through a riptide.

Once the threat passes, special cells in your brain send out an all-clear signal to return your body to normal. This allows your digestive system to return to the business of digesting food, your heart rate and blood pressure to return to calmer levels, and your blood glucose levels to drop (which may leave you a bit light-headed). Essentially, your body is told to relax—the threat is over. If the threat lasted for just a few minutes, then it would take just a few minutes to return your body to normal. But what if you're facing a chronic threat, like a rotten job, overwhelming bills, a bad marriage? That's another story.

Women and stress

For the past 50 years, stress research has focused only on male animals (including men). From these studies, researchers came up with the "fight or flight" catchphrase to explain stress reactions. Then, in 1998, researcher Shelley E. Taylor, Ph.D., decided to study the stress response in female animals. She found that females respond quite differently to non-life-threatening stress, particularly if they're tending young offspring. Turns out female animals don't get nearly as alarmed as their male counterparts. In fact, they are more likely to tend to their young and seek comfort in other females than to either fight or run away. Dr. Taylor went on to test her theory on men and women and found that, in general, men tend to isolate themselves when they feel stressed while women confide their problems to each other. As Dr. Taylor describes it in her book, *The Tending Instinct,* women "tend and befriend."

Chronic stress and IBS

be alert to coping patterns

What happens when a perceived threat lingers for weeks or months? Long-term negative stressors, such as a messy divorce, becoming ill, or getting laid off from work, typically last for months, sometimes years. This means you never get the all-clear signal and your body never gets a chance to return to equilibrium. It's as if your body is in a constant state of alert. Over time, this can take a physical toll, especially if you perceive these stressors as negative. A kind of learned helplessness can set in, a feeling that events are out of your control. This in turn can lead to lowered motivation and self-esteem. Again, perception is key—which is why some people thrive on such stressors as deadlines for a long-term project they're passionate about, while others who don't feel emotionally involved or in control of their work feel anxious and overwhelmed.

When it comes to long-term stress, having a sense of control is crucial. Long-term negative stress can lead to bouts of anxiety, aggression, and depression. Some scientists believe that chronic stress has a harmful effect on the immune system and the endocrine system, making people more vulnerable to illness and infection. Whether you have an illness or not, when it comes to chronic stress you need to work on improving your coping skills.

So, how do you cope with long-term stress? For starters, look at how you have coped in the past with other chronic stressors, especially negative ones. Did you isolate yourself from friends and family? Seek out comfort foods? Sleep a lot? Fall into bad habits, such as smoking or drinking? It's also a good idea to recall how your parents or other significant caregivers handled negative stressors. You may have internalized their coping responses without realizing it.

Negative Coping Responses

There are several negative coping responses that everyone uses at one time or another when dealing with long-term stress. Here's a roundup.

◆ **Deny your problems.** This is a common response for many people—they simply ignore their problems. Or, to take their minds off their problems, they throw themselves into their work or social life.

◆ **Dwell on your problems.** This is usually a learned response. Did your parents or caregivers fret excessively over your health as you were growing up? Or did they ignore your health completely? If they went to either of these extremes, you may find yourself obsessing about your health. If these thoughts become chronic, you should see a therapist who can help you break the pattern of obsessive rumination.

◆ **Procrastinate in decision making.** Instead of thinking through the problem at hand and coming to a decision about what steps to take, you endlessly analyze the situation and talk about the same problem and solution over and over again with friends and family.

◆ **Seek thrills.** Here you look for thrills or experiences to distract you from your problems.

◆ **Get angry and lash out at others.** This is known as displaced aggression. It's when you take out your anger at being ill on others and overreact to their responses.

◆ **Withdraw.** This can take the form of physically or emotionally withdrawing from others. Often people under chronic stress cope by sleeping excessively or simply disengaging from the world.

◆ **Overindulge.** You use food as a drug to mask your fears. Drinking too much alcohol is another way to escape chronic stress, as is smoking too many cigarettes or cigars.

Assault on mind and body

stress can lead to physical ailments

Hundreds of studies show that stress aggravates illness—chronic or episodic, life threatening or curable. Uncontrolled stress can weaken your immune system and make you prone to other health problems, such as colds, flu, general malaise, and fatigue. Other effects of stress:

- Chronic stress can exacerbate or even trigger hair loss, make wounds heal more slowly, and make you prone to such dermatological problems as adult acne, rashes, eczema, and hives.
- High stress can lead to binge eating resulting in obesity, which can lead to a host of other problems such as heart disease and diabetes.
- High stress levels—along with negative emotions—release high levels of the stress hormone cortisol, raising blood pressure and cholesterol.
- High levels of stress can make it difficult to get pregnant or make your partner pregnant, because stress affects reproductive hormones in both men and women.
- Stress often triggers severe gastrointestinal problems, from making symptoms of ulcers worse to aggravating already sensitive bowels.
- Chronic muscle tension due to chronic stress can worsen arthritis flare-ups and lower back problems.
- The chronically stressed can have mild memory loss and problems concentrating or organizing their thoughts.
- Chronic stress tends to make any bad habits worse. Smoking, binge drinking, and drug abuse are all linked to chronic stress.

Right Responses

You swear you're going to have a meltdown the next time someone asks you exactly what IBS is. As an alternative, here's a handy, abbreviated explanation as well as answers to the inevitable questions friends and coworkers will ask.

- IBS is a chronic gastrointestinal condition characterized by abdominal pain, diarrhea and/or constipation, gas, bloating, and fatigue.
- Unfortunately, there is no cure at the moment, but scientists are working on it.
- Although there are many theories as to what causes IBS, no one knows for sure, and there are likely numerous causes.
- No, IBS is not contagious, and yes, women are more likely to have IBS than men.
- IBS is sometimes brought on by a stomach illness like gastritis, which causes the body's digestive system to go awry.
- The symptoms of IBS wax and wane. People with IBS have good days and bad days, also known as flares, in which the symptoms flare up or intensify.
- Stress or problems coping with stress can trigger an IBS episode.
- Yes, it is possible to live well with IBS, with some adjustments.

Smart IBS coping strategies

find positive ways to deal with chronic problems

Having a chronic illness like IBS in which the symptoms can be dormant for days and then suddenly flare up can test your coping reserves. Thus, your old coping standbys may not work for long. The trick to coping with a long-term illness is understanding how to live with it. Since there is as of yet no cure for many chronic illnesses (and in particular, none for IBS), the goal becomes reducing your discomfort and improving your emotional and physical well-being. This means really listening to your symptoms and addressing them. Here are some ways to cope.

Create an IBS retreat. Everyone needs a place of their own to retreat to when the going gets tough. This is especially vital when you feel tired or are having uncomfortable symptoms from IBS. For most, this retreat is the bedroom or bathroom. Stock each with good books and magazines and scented candles. Have a comfortable chair in your bedroom with a good reading light and keep your journal handy.

Get organized. Time management becomes a tool you need to use when you have IBS. Your time and energy are now precious commodities that you shouldn't waste. Learn how to separate the things you really need to do now from those you can spread out over time or delegate to others.

Develop healthy habits. Ironically, people often become healthier once they are diagnosed with health problems. That's because they may stop taking their health for granted, and may turn negative habits into healthy ones, such as quitting smoking.

Make attitude adjustments. Life with any chronic problem can make the world seem like a dour place. Put some humor back into your life. Rent funny movies or read humorous books and magazines.

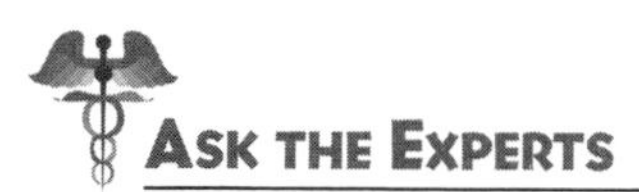

Ask the Experts

I have to travel for work. How can I cut down on stress while I'm on the road?

Traveling is a big stressor, doubly so if you have IBS. That's why it is smart to be proactive and plan ahead. For starters, create a mini-health file with the phone numbers and contact information for all the people on your support team (see Chapter 3). Make sure you bring extra medication just in case (and don't pack it in your luggage; always carry it with you onto the plane or train). Next, don't just pack for your trip. Bring a bit of home with you. Include a pair of comfortable jeans or a favorite shawl. Take along photos of your family to display in your hotel room. Also try a scented candle to get rid of the sterile "hotel" smell. Your goal is to detoxify the stress of travel with things that instantly signal comfort and relaxation.

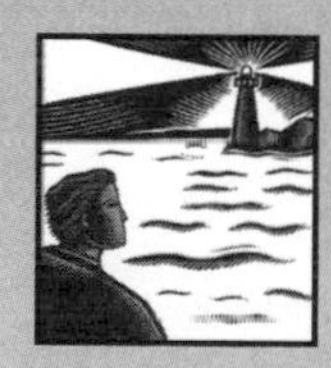

FIRST PERSON INSIGHTS

Chocolate rewards

Ever since my IBS started acting up two years ago, I have dreaded traveling. Unfortunately, it's part of my job. I've managed, but it isn't easy. I now know every rest stop on all the major highways in my state, not to mention where the bathrooms are at all the major airports in the U.S. Because of my IBS, I felt I deserved a reward when I hit the road. So whenever I stopped at rest stops, I would buy my favorite candy bar, something I never let myself eat at home. Then one day I was reading an article about IBS and how chocolate can trigger IBS flare-ups. I started to review my IBS status on my past few trips and wondered if the chocolate was to blame. The next two trips, I laid off all chocolate. Sure enough, I found my symptoms were much better. But what was really surprising was how hard it was to give up that chocolate. I realized then that I had turned it into my very own medication for stress. Now I've come up with a new stress "reward." I get a massage when I come home from each trip.

Sam K., Scottsdale, AZ

Take an IBS stress inventory

how IBS can stress you

No one wants to think their stress levels are out of control, but sometimes you have to confront the stress of a health problem head on, especially if you feel your IBS is overwhelming your life despite treatment. One way is to take a personal stress inventory. Consider the following questions:

- Are you having difficulty accepting a diagnosis of IBS and the fact that there is no cure?
- Are you getting disgusted with trying new medications, none of which seem to work for you?
- Are you spending a lot of time—to the exclusion of all else—researching IBS and other illnesses?
- If your IBS is not responding to treatment, do you hesitate to plan social outings with friends or family because you're afraid of another flare up?

These questions aren't scientific. But they do provide a starting point to assess how the stressors of living with IBS may be affecting you. Again, it doesn't really matter if your symptoms occur once a month, three times a week, or an hour here and there. The point is that you have an extra stress in your life—IBS. If any of these questions seem particularly pertinent to you, talk to your health care professional. He or she may be able to allay some of your fears. A support group (see pages 60–61) may also help by allowing you to share your experiences with others who have IBS. And if no one close to you understands the disease, educate them. Stress is part of life. But the stress of IBS doesn't have to take over your life.

Find Good Listeners

Don't be surprised if, when you mention that you have IBS, your listener immediately cuts you off and tells you about his friend's experience with it. Why does that happen? Well, your friend may be trying to gain a sense of involvement in your plight and show that he has some experience with or knowledge of your situation and that he's capable of understanding your pain. But sometimes it can also be a way to create distance. By telling another person's story, he takes you out of the spotlight and puts his friend in it. This can give him a needed sense of control and distance while he absorbs your news.

Ideally, you want your friends to be good listeners—maybe ask a few questions but still keep the focus on you. Since it can be uncomfortable to hear about a total stranger's problems when you have just revealed your own, tell your friend that you're not ready to talk about your illness in detail. Then change the subject. And, if you don't want your friend to share your news with others, be sure to tell your friend to keep your conversation confidential.

Learning to relax

beat chronic stress at its own game

Our bodies are brilliantly designed to handle stress. They are also designed to handle relaxation. In fact, both the stress response and the relaxation response are hardwired into our brains. Doctors are just now beginning to understand the power of relaxation on the body—both to rejuvenate and to heal.

Think back to a time when you felt truly relaxed. What was going on? You were probably in a quiet, comfortable space where you had no pressures to do anything and could sit back and enjoy the day. You felt peaceful and at one with the world. For most people, that is the definition of a vacation. Here's the news flash: To be healthy, your body needs a little vacation every day. Here's how to get it.

Quiet time. Carve out 10 minutes of the day to simply sit and be quiet. Meditation practices are very helpful in teaching people how to quiet their minds and relax. See pages 182–183 for more on this.

Deep breathing. When you're stressed, your breathing becomes shortened, so much so that you can hyperventilate during acute stress. Counter this natural instinct by purposefully taking four deep breaths every time you feel stressed. Breathe in through your nose, hold the breath for five seconds, then release the air through your mouth.

Exercise. Chronic muscle tension is part and parcel of a chronic stress response. Counteract it by taking a walk or playing a round of tennis. Your goal is to keep your body limber and moving. For a more relaxing exercise, consider taking a class in yoga or tai chi (see pages 190–191 for more information).

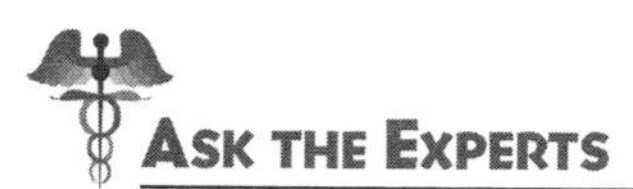

Ask the Experts

I have been anxious for so long, I don't think anything will help. What can I do?

If you've been enduring chronic stressors for a long time, trying to relax overnight isn't going to work. In fact, it will just make you more stressed. You need to retrain your body to feel and behave relaxed. Consider taking a short-term workshop to help you learn how to relax. Or ask your doctor to refer you to a stress clinic or a stress specialist. You can also take courses on stress management. The American Management Association offers two-day workshops on managing stress; call them at 800-262-9699. Or try your local YMCA or YWCA; both usually offer stress management classes.

I hear writing about stressful events helps you get over them. True?

Some studies find that writing about stressful issues or traumatic experiences can help improve the immune system. Use your health journal (see pages 24–25) to write about your concerns.

Getting people to understand

It can be hard to try and explain what it's like to have a chronic health problem to those who have never had one, especially one like IBS where you don't look sick. Try to find an analogy that works. Most working people can relate to the experience of being laid off. In both cases—being laid off and getting IBS—the situation occurs through no fault of your own. After you lose a job, there is a sense of being an outsider—you miss your work routine and feel cut off from the "normal" working world. You are also concerned about your future and anxious to get back to your old life. This is a lot like the experience of having IBS.

Your partner's concerns

how chronic illness can affect relationships

When one half of a couple has an illness, both members usually need to reassess their partnership. If it's a temporary illness, then it's usually a question of juggling practical matters, such as who will pick up the kids while you're sick in bed. But when symptoms are no longer signs of a temporary illness but the manifestation of a lingering health problem, a more in-depth reassessment is needed.

When it comes to handling the ordeals of IBS, couples need to first look at each partner's role and responsibilities in the relationship. Each of you must state what changes you think need to be made. This may mean reassigning roles, be it cleaning duties or paying the bills, when an IBS flare occurs. Often couples fall into the trap of one partner becoming the dominant caregiver and the other becoming the professional patient. Don't let that happen. IBS symptoms wax and wane. You need to work out set plans for the tough times as well as the good.

Not surprisingly, when your symptoms of IBS flare up you are not going to be feeling particularly amorous. Talk about your concerns and listen to your partner. The important thing is to keep the lines of communication open and not to shut down. A good therapist, knowledgeable about the effects of chronic disease on sexuality, may be able to help you work through these issues. To find a therapist for your particular concern, start at the American Association of Sex Educators, Counselors, and Therapists (**www.aasect.org**).

Know Your Enemy

◆ **Know your IBS.** Studies show that people who learn about their condition are most successful in dealing with it. Though the Internet can be fraught with misinformation (see Chapter 9), more than half of patients with chronic illness use the Internet as a source of information, and most find it helpful. Nearly 90 percent, however, say their doctors are the most help, especially if they take the time to explain the illness and what to expect in the future.

◆ **Be aware of depression.** If you're feeling helpless and hopeless, that depressive state can be a real barrier to success. Studies find 9 out of 10 people with IBS are also depressed. Researchers aren't quite sure of the correlation, but they do know one thing: Depression is a problem that needs to be treated. You and your family should be educated about the signs and symptoms of depression and you should let your doctor know if you're experiencing any of them. Conversely, your doctor should also be on the lookout for the signs.

◆ **Get off the couch.** Taking some form of action immediately after a diagnosis seems to provide the best long-term results for living well with a chronic illness. Think about lifestyle changes you may have to make and how you can adapt to these changes. If you avoid the issue, deny the diagnosis, or just withdraw, hoping your illness will disappear, you won't be very successful in dealing with it.

On the job

proper medical care is smart business

Great, you woke up and dressed for work. You are a bit anxious about the presentation you need to make today. After a glass of juice, you head for your car, only to make a dash for the bathroom, where you have terrible diarrhea. More sprints to the bathroom. You are now 30 minutes late to work and your anxiety level is rising with each passing minute.

Sound familiar? If you're a person with IBS, one of the toughest stressors is your job. People miss more days of work due to IBS than the common cold. This fact can be very hard for bosses to understand. They may feel you're shirking your work. You have some options. You can talk to your boss about the nature of IBS. Take heart: Most bosses will try to accommodate you. See if you and your boss can work out a contingency plan if you are too ill to come into the office. For instance, you might see if you can set up a home office and telecommute.

If your boss isn't understanding, or demotes or fires you, you can file a discrimination charge through the Americans with Disabilities Act, or ADA. If you do need to quit work and go on disability, it is vital that you have a doctor who understands IBS and can explain your condition to your disability insurance carrier.

Ask the Experts

I am between jobs and don't have any health insurance right now. How do I find inexpensive health insurance that will cover my IBS?

You should consider health insurance coverage based on membership rather than employment. Consider joining a trade or professional organization that has its own health insurance. For example, if you are a graphic artist, you can join the AIGA, the American Institute of Graphic Artists. It has an insurance plan for its members, and once you join you become eligible for coverage.

I have had to miss a couple of days of a job-related workshop due to an IBS flare-up. Should I tell my boss about my illness?

This is totally up to you. Everyone gets sick from time to time. And we are all entitled to use our sick days as we need them. So, it is not necessary to go public about your health to your employer unless your performance at work is suffering because of it. Only you can know that. However, if you find you need extra sick days because of your IBS, then it might be a good idea to explain your situation to your boss. You may be able to create a flexible schedule to accommodate your needs or perhaps telecommute to work on those days when your IBS is really acting up.

Helpful resources

Instant Relief: Tell Me Where It Hurts and I'll Tell You What to Do
by Peggy W. Brill, P.T., and Susan Suffes

The Relaxation & Stress Reduction Workbook
by Martha Davis, Ph.D., et al

The Chronic Illness Workbook
by Patricia A. Fennel

Managing Stress: Principles and Strategies for Health and Wellbeing (with CD-ROM)
by Brian Luke Seaward, Ph.D.

Mind, Stress, Emotions: The New Science of Mood
by Gene Wallenstein, Ph.D.

Chapter 11

Complementary Therapies

What to expect 174

The complementary approach 176

IBS and stress management 178

Biofeedback 180

Meditation 182

Herbs, vitamins, and minerals 184

Hypnotherapy 186

Acupuncture 188

Yoga, the "mindful" exercise 190

Helpful resources 192

What to expect
identifying your needs

Determining which complementary therapies will work best for you depends on what troubles you most about your irritable bowel syndrome. There are a number of alternative therapies from which to choose, spanning the range from herbs and vitamins to hands-on treatments, such as chiropractic therapy, massage, and acupuncture. Then there are treatments that focus on the mind/body connection, such as biofeedback and meditation, yoga and tai chi.

As you explore complementary therapies, be certain to discuss your plans and discoveries with your doctor. It is essential that she know what you're doing.

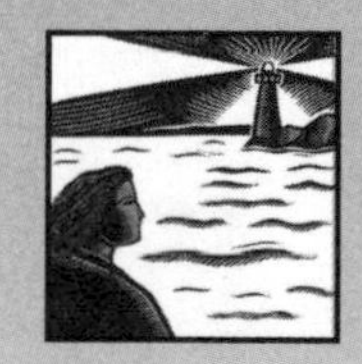

FIRST PERSON INSIGHTS

Buyer beware

I have been dealing with irritable bowel syndrome for five years now. The medication helped, but I was getting fed up with the gas. I was in a health food store and asked the clerk about herbs to help with flatulence. She showed me about six different herbs that are supposed to help. Well, I bought them all. I tried them for a while, but they didn't do much. I mentioned the fact I was taking these pills to my doctor. He wasn't happy that I took the herbs on my own without telling him. He said there can be adverse herb and drug interactions, as well as adverse reactions with other herbs. We sat in his office and went through all the medications I had tried—prescription, over-the-counter, and health food store stuff. He said if I wanted to try something alternative, try biofeedback, but to stay away from herbal supplements unless I talk to him ahead of time.

—Kayla W., New Orleans, LA

◆ **Research what's available.** Support groups can be extremely helpful sources of information. Ask the research librarian at your library to help you. Do an Internet search using the name of your illness plus the name of the therapy you want to explore. For example, irritable bowel syndrome + peppermint oil. (For more information on using the Internet, see Chapter 9.)

◆ **Avoid thinking that because something is "natural" it is benign.** Many of the so-called natural or organic substances touted by alternative healers have not been tested, let alone approved, by the FDA. Testimonials and anecdotal evidence do not make something safe. Be especially wary of taking any products or supplements sold directly by a healer. Talk with your doctor before you try anything.

◆ **Track how you're feeling.** It's tempting to think that you feel lousy all the time. In truth, you have good days and bad days. The more you know about what makes you feel better or worse, the more you can use that knowledge to improve your well-being. Review your health journal (see pages 24–25).

◆ **Bear the expense in mind.** Complementary treatments can cost as much as standard methods—or more, given that insurance doesn't cover most costs. Be as frank with practitioners about your finances as you are about your physical condition. Some practitioners may be willing to negotiate their fees.

◆ **Don't fall for the notion that if the therapy fails, you've failed.** Nothing, not even antibiotics, works equally well for everyone. Give the new therapy a fair trial—some can take a while to show a benefit—but if you're not feeling better, give it up and try something else. Or try seeing another person who practices the same therapy; that person may have an insight that makes all the difference.

The complementary approach

look before you leap

In recent years, patient demand has dictated that medicine become less high tech and more high touch—and the use of nontraditional treatments has steadily risen. In fact, today even the prestigious National Institutes of Health has recognized the trend with its National Center for Complementary and Alternative Medicine (NCCAM). Among its goals are to find out which treatments really do provide relief for various health conditions.

When used alone, these out-of-the-mainstream treatments are often referred to as alternative. When used in addition to conventional medicine, they may be called complementary. According to the National Institutes of Health, the list of what are considered complementary or alternative therapies changes continually as more are proven to be safe and effective and are adopted into conventional health care, and as new approaches to health care emerge.

If you decide to explore complementary therapies, be certain to discuss your plans and discoveries with your doctor. It's essential that your doctor know what you're doing in order to be able to judge how it might interact with your standard treatment.

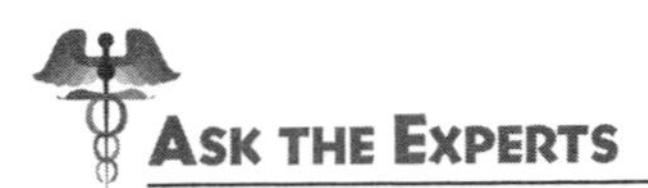

Where do I find alternative practitioners?

The National Center for Complementary and Alternative Medicine (NCCAM) suggests you contact a professional organization for the type of practitioner you are seeking. Often these organizations provide referrals to practitioners as well as information about the therapy. You can find them by searching the Internet or through directories in libraries (ask the librarian). One such directory is the Directory of Health Organizations Online (DIRLINE), **http://nlm.nih.gov/**, compiled by the National Library of Medicine. It contains locations and descriptive information about a variety of alternative health organizations.

What happens if my regular doctor says no to anything alternative?

First, most physicians recognize that their patients often seek alternative treatments without informing them. Your doctor will probably be happy that you're even discussing the concept before plunging ahead. If your doctor says no without giving you a reason other than it's all a "bunch of baloney," you need to weigh that position against your own desire to try something new. Keep in mind that the treatment may or may not help your IBS, and might even harm you.

It also depends on what treatment you're seeking. Some treatments are baloney, some aren't, and some have very good studies behind them. Chances are good, though, that your physician will respect your desire for a remedy, regardless of where it comes from. Whatever you do, be sure to keep your doctor informed.

IBS and stress management

teaching your mind to soothe your body

As you know, stress is a major trigger for your IBS symptoms. So learning to control and better cope with the stress in your life helps minimize your symptoms. That's where mind/body modalities come in. They teach you to be more conscious of stress and give you practical things to do about it. With proper guidance, stress management techniques can yield enormous benefits, not just physically, but also mentally, emotionally, and spiritually. Relaxation therapy encompasses a wide range of techniques designed to reduce stress and tension. Some of the more popular ones follow.

Progressive muscle relaxation. You do this by systematically tensing and relaxing the muscles in each part of your body. While sitting comfortably or lying down, inhale and clench your facial muscles, hold the tension for a moment, then exhale and relax those muscles. Do the same thing with your shoulders, one arm, then the other, and so on, through your body until you get to your toes. When you're done, stay quietly where you are and breathe normally for a few minutes.

Guided imagery. The idea here is to imagine a peaceful place and put yourself in the scene. This can be done with a partner who provides the "guidance" by describing the scene, but you can also do all the imagining yourself or listen to a narrated audiotape, soothing music, or environmental sounds, such as birdsongs or ocean waves.

Deep breathing. You wouldn't think breathing could make such a difference in your stress levels, but it does. Taking a few minutes each day to practice slow, deep breathing can help relieve stomach pain as well as improve mental sharpness. Start by standing, sitting, or lying still. Place one hand on your belly and slowly inhale until you feel your hand rise and your lungs are full (your belly should expand); then exhale slowly and completely. Repeat that for 10 or 12 breaths. Some people find it energizing to do this type of deep breathing before they get out of bed in the morning.

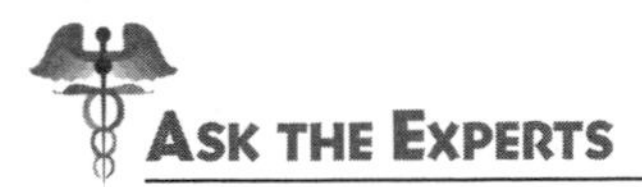

Ask the Experts

Why do people always tell me to breathe deeply whenever I get stressed or upset or angry?

When you get upset, it is usually because something did not go your way or something happened that was out of your control. Most of us respond to such uncomfortable situations by taking lots of shallow breaths. This can be especially harmful for those with IBS, because short shallow breathing leads to lots of swallowed air, which in turn leads to gas. In fact, some people use their breath as a barameter of how they are feeling. The more stressed they are, the more shallow their breathing.

One way to counteract feelings of stress or fear is to do something that you *can* control, namely, change your breathing pattern. By concentrating on your breath and inhaling deeply (your belly should expand) and exhaling slowly, you are not only getting more oxygen into your blood, but also telling yourself that, despite all else, you are in control.

Biofeedback

learning to control the pain

Biofeedback is one of the most effective therapies for chronic health conditions. And because of its success, many experts don't even consider biofeedback an alternative approach but an integrated component of their treatment plans. The National Institutes of Health considers biofeedback to be mainstream medicine and recommends its greater use.

Biofeedback works on the principle that you can be taught to control certain body processes that seem to happen on their own, like heart rate, skin temperature, brain waves, and of course, digestion. To get the information—the feedback—that will allow you to learn to change the way your mind/body system responds to stress and pain, such as blood-vessel dilation and muscle tension, the biofeedback practitioner uses small sensors usually placed on the hands, shoulders, or scalp. These sensors are connected to a computer. Depending on which sensors are attached, the computer transforms the information it receives and makes it visible or audible via the monitor or speakers. This allows you to see or hear your breath rate, pulse rate, skin temperature and conductance, even your brain waves, live and in color!

You are then taught how to breathe more deeply or asked to visualize a relaxing scene, both of which influence the sensor readings and what you hear or see via the computer. During a training session, you practice various relaxation techniques while getting continuous feedback from the sensors. Thus, you can see how relaxed breathing can lower your pulse rate or change your brain waves. And you see how sensitive your body is to stressful thinking.

After several sessions, you should be able to consciously exert greater control over your mind/body responses and see and feel the changes as your hands warm, your muscles relax, your breath slows and deepens, and your mind relaxes.

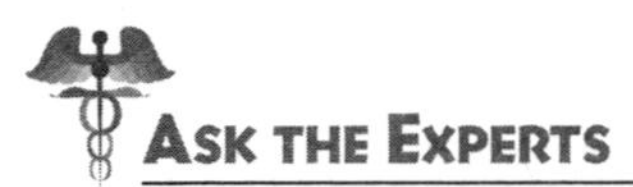

Ask the Experts

Why are sensors placed on the hands?

Skin temperature and skin conductance are usually measured on the fingers. The sweat glands and the blood flow through the hands are especially sensitive to stress and emotional reactivity. The stress response lowers peripheral blood flow, which makes hands and feet feel cold, thus the expression "getting cold feet." When you learn how to relax profoundly, your hand temperature rises and skin conductance drops. Over time, you can learn to sustain a lower level of stress and reactivity throughout the day.

How do you teach your brain to change its waves?

The basic principle in all biofeedback is that once you can perceive something, you can begin to change it. The computer makes your brain waves appear before you, linked to a graph or a game like a maze. At the beginning of the maze is a blinking light. If your brain is producing the selected brain waves, you can power that blinking light to race through the maze. The blinking stops when your brain moves out of the selected zone. Depending on which brain waves are being trained to increase or decrease, this method can help people learn how to focus their thinking and can lower tension throughout the body, which in turn results in better digestion and less pain.

Where can I find a biofeedback practitioner?

The best place to look is the Internet. Check out the Biofeedback Certification Institute of America at **www.bcia.org** or the Association for Applied Psychophysiology & Biofeedback at **www.aapb.org**. Both sites have tabs to help you find a practitioner in your area.

Meditation

using the metaphysical to help the physical

Studies show that regular meditation can lower blood pressure, relieve chronic pain, and reduce cortisol levels, a hormonal measure of the body's stress. It may also help if you suffer from irritable bowel syndrome because it teaches your body how to relax. Dr. Herber Benson, a Harvard cardiologist, did a great deal of research on meditation and found that regular meditation can actually lower autonomic nervous system activity—meaning that meditation allows your body to truly relax. He dubbed this phenomenon the relaxation response.

Subsequent studies on meditation and IBS found that, practiced regularly, meditation and relaxation improved symptoms and enabled people with the condition to cope better in their daily lives.

How can something as simple as meditation perform such wonders? There is no hard answer. Most practitioners say it works because it transports both the body and the mind into a uniquely unified state. As meditation teacher Dr. Lawrence Edwards explains, "Meditation is a transformation process. Over time, meditation evolves into a process where you feel a sense of peace and inner freedom. Every time you meditate, you are increasing the reservoir of meditative power that you can tap into during stressful or challenging moments."

There are a number of different meditation techniques to consider. Some focus on the breath, requiring you to simply observe yourself breathing in and out; others use a **mantra** (a special word or phrase) that is repeated over and over again. The goal is the same: to focus your attention away from the thoughts whirling around inside your head. The repetition of breath or mantra helps calm the mind so it can enter into a meditative state. It may be helpful to light a scented candle or burn incense. That's because your mind will associate the fragrance with relaxation, registering that it's time to settle down. It's also helpful to meditate at the same time every day and for the same amount of time, even if it's only for a few minutes.

How to Meditate

- Find a place where you can sit quietly without interruption for 20 minutes.
- Sit comfortably, but keep your back erect—this will help support alertness and open breathing. (You can meditate lying down if you are not able to sit up.)
- Set a timer for 15 to 20 minutes.
- Close your eyes and bring your attention to your breathing. Focus on the movement of your diaphragm as you inhale and exhale.
- As you settle into this quiet breathing, you can silently repeat your mantra or any word you wish. You can use the traditional Sanskrit words *om namah shivaya,* or silently say a phrase of your own choosing, or simply use the words "one, two, three, four."
- When your mind begins to wander, as it inevitably will, just gently return your focus to your breath or mantra. This pattern of wandering and returning is the beginning of teaching your mind to let go of its worries.
- When the timer buzzes, notice how peaceful you feel.
- Open your eyes and stretch.
- Choose a regular time and place to meditate. Start by meditating for 20 minutes three times a week. Stay with it.

Herbs, vitamins, and minerals

nature's medicine chest

There are several herbs and botanicals associated with irritable bowel syndrome relief. If you are considering taking any herbal supplement, you should first check with your doctor. Sometimes herbs, even vitamins and minerals, can interact with over-the-counter or prescription drugs that you're taking. Plus, the FDA regulates neither herbs nor vitamins. That means it is difficult to know the quantity and quality of the supplement you're taking.

Still, there have been a few studies on supplements and vitamins for irritable bowel syndrome. Here's what seems to work best.

Aloe. Aloe is commonly used in IBS, primarily to treat constipation. There aren't many studies on aloe in IBS, but one found that a combination of aloe vera, celandine (a member of the buttercup family), and psyllium (fiber) improved symptoms more than a placebo, or pretend treatment. Aloe can trigger diarrhea in some people, so monitor your body's reactions carefully and discontinue use if diarrhea results.

Peppermint oil. Also called *Mentha piperita*, peppermint is a traditional folk remedy used for thousands of years as a means of diminishing gas (that's why restaurants put peppermints by their front doors). Its effects on IBS are not just folkloric, however, but scientific, with numerous studies finding that peppermint oil extract (available in health food stores) reduces the gas and bloating associated with IBS. It is also often combined with caraway oil, which seems to improve its effectiveness. If you have GERD or acid reflux, you should avoid peppermint oil, since it also relaxes the lower esophageal sphincter, which can worsen reflux symptoms.

Chinese medicine. You'll need to see a practitioner skilled in using Chinese herbal remedies for this, but several studies point to success with traditional Chinese medicine in treating IBS. IBS is often treated with medicines called Curing Pills, which contain about 15 different herbal remedies, and a tea of Shen Qu Cha.

Psyllium seed husk. This natural laxative, which helps bring on normal bowel activity in some people with IBS, improved IBS symptoms in well-designed clinical studies. Note: Psyllium husks are the active ingredient in several over-the-counter fiber supplements, such as Metamucil.

Other herbs worth considering

Primrose oil. This remedy is often used to help women with hormonally related conditions. One study of women whose IBS got worse during and before their periods found that taking enough evening primrose oil to provide 360 to 400 mg of gamma linolenic acid (GLA) per day improved symptoms in more than half the women studied.

Grapefruit seed extract. One small study found 150 mg of encapsulated grapefruit seed extract (GSE) three times a day improved symptoms in study participants.

Hypnotherapy

more than just a party game

One of the most exciting complementary treatments for IBS is hypnotherapy, which numerous well-designed studies have found to be effective. One study had 204 people with IBS undergo 12 weekly hypnotherapy sessions, then followed these participants for six years. Seven out of 10 reported that their symptoms initially improved, and of those, 8 out of 10 found they felt better for at least 5 years. Additionally, participants saw their doctors less often and used less medication after undergoing hypnotherapy.

While you might think of hypnosis as some kind of parlor trick or mind control, it's actually a very well respected medical treatment, its use significantly growing over the past 20 years. In fact, studies find it works for everything from pain management to allergy and asthma control to helping surgical wounds heal faster. Even the American Medical Association approved of its use as early as 1958.

The core of hypnotherapy lies in the complex connection between the mind and the body. Like biofeedback, hypnotherapy deliberately harnesses the power of the mind to affect the physical systems in the body. In fact, researchers find that parts of the brain become more active during hypnosis, with one study indicating that during hypnosis for pain the prefrontal cortex of the brain, which controls concentration, directs other areas of the brain to reduce or eliminate their awareness of pain.

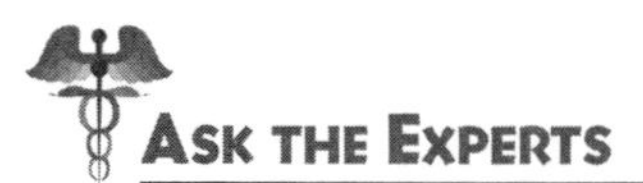

Ask the Experts

I'm worried that if I undergo hypnosis for my IBS, I'll do something silly or lose control.

Trained hypnotherapists use various methods to help their patients access the trance state. Which approach they use depends on your individual personality and needs. And, contrary to popular perceptions about hypnosis, you don't "lose control" when hypnotized and you can't be made to do things you wouldn't normally do. Plus, you don't lose consciousness or develop amnesia. In fact, in many ways it's similar to meditation, visualization, and deep breathing. Once you're relaxed, the therapist provides suggestions, helping you visualize your body working in a different manner.

How do I find a good hypnotherapist?

Your best bet for finding a medical hypnotherapist isn't the yellow pages; it's online at the following professional associations:

The American Psychotherapy & Medical Hypnosis Association
www.apmha.com
The association, which promotes the ethical use of hypnosis, offers certification to medical providers who have completed a six- to eight-week training course.

The American Society of Clinical Hypnosis
www.asch.net
The largest U.S. organization for health and mental health care professionals using clinical hypnosis, the ASCH also offers a certification program.

Acupuncture

help for IBS

There is no published evidence yet to support the use of acupuncture for IBS. But this ancient therapy, which arose in China more than 2,000 years ago, is slowly gaining ground. Acupuncture involves placing fine needles at specific points on the body's surface. According to a 1998 consensus statement from the National Institutes of Health, acupuncture is clearly useful for adults with postoperative and chemotherapy nausea and vomiting, as well as (probably) the nausea of pregnancy. In addition, the NIH states that there is promising evidence suggesting that the technique can help addiction, stroke rehabilitation, migraine headaches, fibromyalgia, osteoarthritis, lower back pain, carpal tunnel syndrome, asthma, and other problems.

Approximately 9 to 12 million Americans turn to acupuncture each year for relief from chronic medical ailments. But acupuncture isn't a cure-all. It is best used for people with chronic, long-standing pain problems—such as musculoskeletal disorders—and for those with nonchronic conditions such as pain related to injuries and other traumas.

Traditional Chinese practitioners believe acupuncture unblocks and balances the energy, or chi (sometimes spelled qi), flowing through your body along pathways called meridians. If the flow of chi is blocked or unbalanced at any point in a pathway, illness may result (according to the belief).

Western practitioners who have studied acupuncture theorize that it reduces pain through blocked biological mechanisms possibly involving opioid peptides (the body's own painkillers) and stimulation of the hypothalamus and pituitary gland, or changes in neurotransmitters, hormones, or immune function.

Ask the Experts

How deep are the acupuncture needles inserted?

Only a few millimeters. The needles are very fine, and discomfort is minimal.

If I use acupuncture, do I need anything else?

Generally, acupuncture is not used as a stand-alone therapy. Practitioners certified in acupuncture may also recommend some herbal treatments, for example.

How do I find a practitioner?

Again, talk to your doctor. Most, but not all, states provide licensing or registration for physician and nonphysician acupuncturists. If possible, check to see if your practitioner is certified by the National Certification Commission for Acupuncture and Oriental Medicine. Physicians who use acupuncture in their practices are generally certified by the American Academy of Medical Acupuncture.

Yoga, the "mindful" exercise

using yoga to help you handle your pain

Yoga teaches you to stay alert to your body as you exercise and to coordinate your breathing with your movements. For these reasons, many people consider yoga a "mindful" exercise, a form of meditation in motion. But how does that help your IBS?

Studies have shown that yoga has a strong antidepressant effect and that it promotes mental and emotional clarity; improves balance, flexibility, strength, and stamina; relieves chronic muscle aches; eliminates stress; and helps regulate your metabolism. All exercise helps improve circulation, and that in turn can help stave off some of the complications of IBS. Yoga is especially helpful when used in combination with aerobic exercise, such as brisk walking or bike riding, and traditional strength building, such as working out with light weights.

Yoga is taught in many different ways. Some classes are slow paced; others are as lively as a step-aerobics class, so shop around until you find something that suits you. Typically, yoga classes can be paid for one at a time, or in sets of 5 or 10 with a discounted price. Some health clubs offer yoga classes, often at no additional cost to the membership price.

If you're curious but skeptical, ask to observe a class. Talk to your yoga teacher about specific poses that can help with abdominal pain, gas, bloating, diarrhea, or constipation. A well-trained teacher should be able to point you in the right direction. Once you know the proper poses, you can do them on your own at home. This is welcome news for many with IBS, who don't feel up to leaving their home during flare-ups.

Qigong and Tai Chi

According to the National Qigong Association, qigong is "an ancient Chinese health care system that integrates physical postures, breathing techniques, and focused intention." Pronounced "CHEE-gung"—and sometimes spelled ChiKung—the word means "cultivating energy."

Tai chi is a form of qigong; both are practiced for health maintenance, healing, and increased vitality. Tai chi is also a martial art and helps prepare the person, mentally and physically, for fighting. Both qigong and tai chi consist of a series of dancelike gestures that are performed in a specific sequence. The sequence of gestures is called a form, and there are long and short forms of the exercises. In tai chi, the short form takes about 10 minutes to complete; it's a bit longer for qigong. Practitioners of the form say that the sense of vitality you feel afterward will last throughout the day. As with yoga, once you have learned the forms in the proper sequence, you can practice them at home. This has been a real boon for those who want to keep up their exercise routines but, due to an IBS flare-up, don't feel comfortable leaving home and being too far away from a bathroom.

Helpful resources

Beyond the Relaxation Response: How to Harness the Healing Power of Your Personal Beliefs
by Herbert Benson, M.D.

IBS Breakthrough: Healing Irritable Bowel Syndrome for Good with Chinese Medicine
by Leigh Fortson and Bing Lee

National Center for Complementary and Alternative Medicine (NCCAM) located at the National Institutes of Health, Bethesda, MD
This government agency provides information about and sponsors research in complementary therapies.
888-644-6226
www.nccam.nih.gov

American Council on Science and Health
212-362-7044
www.acsh.org

Complementary and Alternative Healing University
This site is full of advice and explanations about every kind of alternative treatment under the sun.
www.alternativehealing.org

American College for the Advancement of Medicine
This organization is an excellent resource for finding alternative, licensed doctors practicing in your area.
800-532-3688
www.acam.org

Chapter 12

The New Normal

Life with IBS	194
Stages of adjustment	196
Beyond acceptance	198
Beginning the journey	200
Talking about it	202
Creating a new life	204
Helpful resources	206

Life with IBS

it can be a rocky road

In your not-too-distant past, whenever you got sick you went to a doctor, got a prescription, felt better, and went on with your life. But IBS—despite modern medicine's best efforts—defies this pattern. Sure, there are treatments that can provide relief, but there is no known cure. The reality is that for you now, having IBS is your "new normal."

Unlike other major changes in your life, such as switching careers or getting married, you did not choose to have to adjust to life with IBS. And that lack of choice can make it rough going. But you are not alone. So many people have the condition—or symptoms similar to the ones that you have—that it has become something of a national epidemic. Some researchers estimate that one out of five adults in the United States has IBS.

Actually, a diagnosis of a nonterminal illness like IBS can be a relief. After all, who wouldn't be happy to know they don't have a degenerative illness or some kind of stomach cancer? But that euphoria can be short-lived and is by no means a universal reaction. Many people are overcome with sadness. Others may become angry. The problem is that IBS is not so much a medical disorder as it is a social disabler—it can and does change the way you lead your life. That's because there is no predicting those days when you will need to have ready access to a bathroom.

Because of the social curtailing that can happen with IBS, many people undergo a great many emotional reactions, much like the stages of grief. In fact, you are grieving over your lost way of life. Gone are the days and nights when you could take your need to use the facilities for granted. Now, just going out to the grocery store can become a problem because of the need to have immediate access to a bathroom.

One of the aspects of IBS that can be very difficult to handle is its invisibility. The pain is real, but there are no outward signs of IBS. It's not like walking around with a broken leg. Or even coping with a life-threatening illness like cancer. All your friends and family know is that you are canceling yet another event or outing because of this thing called IBS. This can be extremely frustrating to deal with on a continuous basis.

There will also be a lack of consistency in your symptoms that makes adjusting to IBS particularly hard. The symptoms come and go. Some days are worse than others, some are better. Conversely, it's hard for people to truly understand how you can be fine for weeks at a time, and then miss days of work or a social activity because you've had a flare-up. That unpredictability can make both you and your family anxious. Most people are great at rallying around people in an emergency. They're not that good with painful symptoms that strike at will and continue indefinitely.

Considering these factors, it's not surprising that you feel there's a lack of understanding around you. That's why even during the best of times, you need to talk about your feelings. That's doubly true with IBS because it is a condition that involves many taboo subjects, such as diarrhea and gas. Living with IBS requires an ongoing search for a positive quality of life. Try to keep these two goals in mind: dealing effectively with the symptoms and coping with the way IBS affects your life and lifestyle.

Stages of adjustment

from shock to acceptance

Researchers have learned that the ways in which you cope with the news of any health problem affects your long-term physical and emotional health. They compare your reaction to the five stages of grief, as defined by Dr. Elisabeth Kübler-Ross in her groundbreaking work, *On Death and Dying*. Examine these stages to see where you are. You may not encounter all of them; they are simply a blueprint of how most people respond to loss—be it of a loved one or of their own health.

Denial

It can be tough to make such lifestyle adjustments as taking medication and changing your diet, especially if you have severe IBS. That's why many people try to deny their suffering, hoping it just goes away. It's hard to deal with the loss of personal power and of self-esteem, as well as a loss of independence as your IBS inevitably interferes with your life. Better to just ignore it. But often this type of denial can interfere with treatment and so you don't see your doctor for a new treatment plan because it all seems futile, or so you think. This means you deny any potential new problems as well as the old ones.

What to do? Think through the situation. What would you tell a friend who was experiencing new symptoms, such as severe stomach cramps? Probably the same thing your family and friends are telling you. Seek help. Don't self-diagnose, and don't deny.

Anger, depression, and bargaining

In the first of these three stages, you're mad at everything and everyone: "I see my doctor for checkups. I give to animal welfare groups. I am a good person. This just isn't fair!" Your friends, family, and colleagues act as if your IBS isn't any big deal. You know you don't have a serious illness with a capital S, and you're not going to die from this thing—but in addition to feeling angry, you're likely to be depressed, because no one seems to understand what you're going through and nothing you do makes the IBS go away for good. Lastly, you may even want to bargain your way out of IBS. "If I rest a lot and eat only organic foods, I'll get well."

What to do? You will have to remind yourself that you'll have some great days and some not-so-great days, and that there is rarely such a thing as total recovery. IBS is still with you daily, because there is no cure. It's particularly important to remember that, contrary to what's commonly believed, the majority of people living with chronic illnesses are not elderly or disabled. More than half are between the ages of 18 and 64, and few report that they limit their activities solely based on their disease.

Acceptance

Having gone through some or all of the previous stages, you now accept your IBS as part of yourself, a reality to be lived with, not escaped. You recognize that your best chance for future happiness lies in your understanding of the condition and in your disciplined commitment to staying informed and managing your symptoms.

Beyond acceptance

your job now is to re-create your life

Learning to accept a chronic disorder as part of your life is not easy. You miss the old carefree you. You miss not having to think about where the next bathroom is on a Saturday drive through the country. You now fully understand why your grandparents used to say, "Don't take your health for granted."

Yes, you have this disorder, but it is treatable and it doesn't have to define who you are. You are still you—just a bit different due to your IBS. Yes, it is a different life than the one you had originally planned, before you encountered this problem, but you are learning to accept that. The point is to work with this new reality and make it your own. Here are some helpful suggestions.

Learn about your condition.

Becoming a student of IBS can be an important way to know what is going on with your body. Use as many sources as you can to gather information so you understand what your doctor is doing to help you. Learn about your medications and watch for their side effects. Follow your doctor's instructions and keep focused on the goal—managing your symptoms. Just a word of caution: In this information age, it is easy to access knowledge, but not all the information you access is accurate. Always discuss "new" breakthroughs in IBS with your doctor.

Take control.

The most successful people who have IBS are those who are active participants in their own treatment. This means taking your health in your own hands. How does that work? For starters, it means you choose who treats you. If you like your current doctor, great. But if you feel you aren't getting enough attention from your doctor, then you can change and should change your doctor. The point is to take responsibility, along with your doctor for managing your IBS. It means complying with treatments, and diets you don't understand. And that also means asking questions about treatments and diets you don't understand. The bottom line: Be involved.

Find the right doctor.

In the beginning, it's extremely important to find the right doctor. Don't be afraid to insist on a doctor who understands you and communicates clearly. After all, this is the person who will help you regain your life. You need to have a good relationship, so find someone who will collaborate with you and take an interest in you and your care.

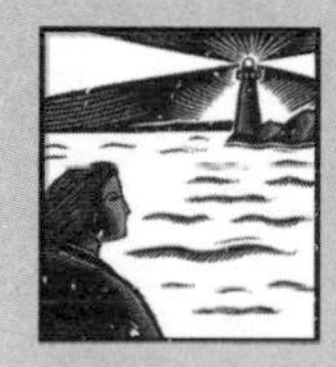

FIRST PERSON INSIGHTS

First me, then them

I think you have to be okay with the invisibility of IBS yourself before you can expect others to accept or understand it. When I was diagnosed with IBS four years ago, my two elementary age sons started acting out and really fighting with each other. Maybe it was because I couldn't stay on top of all their skirmishes like I did in the past. It was quite an adjustment for them as I made subtle changes in how much I allowed myself to be on top of every little thing in their lives, from who got the last dessert to how neatly they did their homework.

Actually, it was an adjustment for all of us. Yet over time, and after plenty of discussions, everyone in the family has come to accept this illness as a part of who I am, to understand that this is how our family now functions. My sons know that when I am resting or in the bathroom, they need to be quiet and not fight. Overall, they manage quite well. I think it has taught them to be more compassionate people.

—Terry G., Indianapolis, IN

Beginning the journey

taking it step by step

After any diagnosis, no one knows what the final outcome will be. It's hard to live with this new, and constant, level of uncertainty and ambiguity. But how you cope and live with this can make all the difference. What seems undoable and unmanageable is really quite doable.

To combat the chaos, follow a few smart strategies. First, get as much information as possible. Understanding the facts can help relieve your anxiety and reduce the fear of the unknown. Besides, knowledge helps you regain control and make informed decisions.

Identify and avoid vicious cycles

For example, having diarrhea from IBS may make you feel discouraged, and being discouraged may contribute to feelings of uselessness. These feelings, in turn, can contribute to a sense of fatigue, which then may increase the feeling of being useless and unhappy. This is a classic vicious cycle.

Be positive

Trying to figure out new ways to enjoy old activities is fine, but if you feel depressed it also helps to focus on things you still do well. Remember that you are a competent, unique person—with many talents and attributes that are still yours.

- Use laughter and humor to reduce stress.
- Build on the talents and activities you can still enjoy.
- Pay attention to your body. How does it feel? How is it reacting to the things you are doing right now? Plan your day accordingly.
- Learn more about yourself. What makes you tense?
- Stick to your goals. They should not diminish because you have IBS.

Educate

Teach your family, friends, and coworkers about IBS. Talk to your family about what you need, what you expect from treatment, and what to do if those meds don't work on occasion.

Get help

Find other people who have IBS. Though friends, coworkers, and family members can be sympathetic, no one knows the pain of IBS better than those who live with it. There are many support groups online, and there may be some "live" support groups in your area. Check out local hospitals to see if they offer IBS support.

Talking about it

learn to talk about your needs

For many people, talking about IBS is embarrassing. They don't want talk about "bathroom stuff." And so they say nothing. If this sounds familiar, then it's time to learn how to talk about having IBS. (Children, especially, need to know that parents suffering from IBS are okay.) Here are a few tips to make it easier.

Pick the time and place to talk. You should feel in control of the conversation. One way to do that is to choose the time and location. Don't get backed into talking about your IBS when you are not ready or not feeling up to it.

Think about what you're going to say. Start by defining the disorder. Explain that while there is no known cause for it, there is treatment. (If you are talking to children, be sure to mention that IBS is not contagious.) Talk about how IBS comes and goes, and then explain how IBS affects you on a day-to-day basis. You might want to list three things your family or friends can do to help you during difficult IBS flare-ups, such as helping with chores or giving you time to be alone or understanding why you have to cancel a social engagement at the last minute. If you are shy, practicing the words ahead of time can help you overcome shyness.

Set the terms and limits of the information you want to share. Your friends and family don't have to know every intimate detail of your struggle with IBS. Tell them what you want to tell them, and don't feel compelled to answer invasive questions. Simply call a halt to the questions and say you don't feel comfortable answering them right now. Also, be sure to state that you don't want this information shared if that is your wish.

Five Rules for Not Talking About Your Illness

1. "How are you?" is a greeting, not a request for medical news. Just because you have a chronic illness, there is no reason to change your usual response. Wait until someone asks specifically about your illness before telling her about it.

2. Fit the answer to your audience. Have a short version and a long version ready. Your spouse may want to hear every detail the minute you come home from your doctor's visit. But your colleagues want only a summarized version.

3. Watch for eyes glazing over. Someone has asked about your illness and seems really interested. So you launch into the long version. Watch for signs of boredom. Does she fidget? Glance around? If you pause or ask a question, is there a slight delay before you have her attention again?

4. After three minutes, change the subject. Even the most loving friend may not be able to take in every detail of an extended medical report. Give her a break. If someone is really interested, she'll return to the subject.

5. Use humor. Have a couple of jokes handy to break up your monologue, or provide an exit line.

Creating a new life

it's time to create a new life

If you take a good look at your life now and the life you led before you got IBS, you are likely to see some differences. It's been a gradual process of cutting out certain foods that don't agree with your stomach as well as cutting back on stresses that trigger your IBS symptoms. In a sense, it is a process of learning how to take care of your stomach by learning to say no to things that aggravate it. But here's the rub—just when you think you have figured out your IBS and you're free of symptoms, it starts up again for no reason that you know. While you may feel you are starting all over again, take heart. You have learned a great deal about IBS and your body's personal reaction to it. If there is one good thing about IBS, it's that it teaches you about your gut and what it needs. And when it comes to chronic conditions like IBS, this means paying continuous attention to your digestion, your emotions, your food choices, your stress levels—anything that can affect your health.

Having a chronic condition like IBS calls for a different way of looking at your health. It is no longer this static thing you can automatically rely upon. Your health is now something that you need to manage on a daily basis. It may take some time to reach this point of acceptance and make peace with something as uncomfortable as IBS. How you ultimately choose to approach the new life that IBS has thrust upon you—and everyone will find their own way—will determine how well you cope and even how good you feel.

Becoming an Advocate

Ways you can give back. There may come days when you have no choice but to ask for help while you are laid up with an IBS flare. In time, many people with IBS learn that there is nothing kinder and more loving than accepting help freely given. Small wonder that people who have undergone physical and emotional trials are the ones who give back to others who are in need.

How can you help those with IBS? You can go online and add your knowledge to the various support groups on the Internet that provide so much help to those in the throes of early diagnosis (see pages 150–151 for Web addresses). You can also join the various nonprofit organizations that support IBS research. Consider volunteering to help with their work. Becoming an advocate is a great way to help others newly diagnosed with IBS.

Helpful resources

The Chronic Illness Workbook
by Patricia A. Fennell

On Death and Dying
by Elisabeth Kübler-Ross, M.D.

Gut Wisdom: Understanding and Improving Your Digestive Health
by Alyce M. Sorokie

Illness as Metaphor
by Susan Sontag

On Being Ill
by Virginia Woolf

Recrafting a Life: Solutions for Chronic Pain and Illness
by Charlie Johnson and Denise Webster

Glossary

abdomen The portion of the human torso above the pelvis and below the diaphragm (*ab*, below; *domen*, the dome). The abdomen contains the stomach, large and small intestines, liver, gallbladder, pancreas, and spleen.

acetylcholine A neurotransmitter active in the transmission of nerve impulses in the parasympathetic branch of the autonomic nervous system.

achalasia The medical term used to describe the failure of the lower esophageal sphincter to relax.

acid reflux disorder Regurgitation of stomach acid into the esophagus. A common cause of heartburn, chest pain, and esophagitis. Also called gastroesophageal reflux disease (GERD), reflux esophagitis.

adhesion An abnormal fibrous band that binds together internal parts (such as organs) that normally are separate. May arise as a consequence of surgery; if causing pain or intestinal obstruction, may be treated surgically.

aerophagia Habitually swallowing air. Ingestion of air.

afferent nerves Nerve fibers that send information to the brain and spinal cord or to the information processing centers of the enteric nervous system (located in the walls of the digestive tract). See also: efferent nerves.

aganglionosis The absence of nerve cells (ganglia).

alimentary canal The route that food follows from the mouth through the various digestive and elimination organs to the anus.

amylase A digestive enzyme that helps to break complex carbohydrates into simpler nutrients.

anal fissure A crack or break in the skin near the anus.

anemia A condition of an insufficient quantity of red blood cells, or of a deficient quality of those cells.

anus The opening of the rectum that allows the ejection of stool.

arteriosclerosis A condition in which the arterioles (small artcrics) thicken and lose elasticity, impeding blood flow. Also called hardening of the arteries.

autonomic nervous system The portion of the nervous system that works automatically, without conscious control. This system has two parts: the sympathetic and parasympathetic nervous systems.

barium A soft, alkaline metal. The insoluble form, barium sulfate, is impervious to X-rays. Crushed and suspended in a solution, barium sulfate can be administered orally or via enema to coat the organs of the alimentary canal and aid in X-ray and fluoroscopic examination. See also: barium enema, upper GI series.

barium enema The medical name for a lower GI (gastrointestinal) test. In this test, barium sulfate is administered via an enema, and the colon and lower portions of the small intestine (the jejunum and ileum) are examined with X-rays or a fluoroscope. See also: barium, upper GI series.

belching Expelling stomach gas from the mouth and nose. Also called eructation.

beta-blocker A colloquial name for beta-adrenergic blocking agents such as propranolol. These drugs inhibit the activity of the sympathetic nervous system and certain hormones, and help relieve the symptoms of irritable bowel syndrome.

bile Produced in the liver and stored in the gallbladder until needed, bile aids the digestion and absorption of dietary fats and stimulates peristalsis.

biliary tract The organs that store and secrete bile (primarily the gallbladder and liver) and the ducts that deliver it to the duodenum.

biopsy A small piece of tissue extracted for diagnostic purposes. The tissue may be extracted by suction with a fine needle or during a surgery.

biopsychosocial model An approach to medicine that considers the influence of biological, psychological, and social (personal and environmental) factors on illness and healing.

bolus The mass of chewed food that is ready to be swallowed or that is in the esophagus en route to the stomach.

borborygmi Audible rumbling, gurgling, splashing sound caused by gas bubbling with liquid in the intestines. Absence of these normally heard sounds may indicate a bowel obstruction.

bowel An informal term for the intestines.

bulking agent A substance that absorbs water in the intestinal tract and increases the size of the stool. Bulky stool stimulates peristalsis and helps relieve constipation. See also: Fiber.

cathartic See: laxative.

celiac disease Also called gluten intolerance, celiac disease is the inability to digest and absorb gliaden, a protein found in grains (wheat, barley, rye, oats). Its symptoms include diarrhea, malnutrition, bleeding tendency, and abnormally low blood calcium (hypocalcemia).

cholecystectomy Surgery to remove the gallbladder. (The prefix cholecyst- means gallbladder.)

cholecystogram An X-ray of the gallbladder.

cholecystokinin A hormone secreted by the duodenum. It stimulates gallbladder contraction and secretion of pancreatic enzymes.

chyme The substance that results when food is mixed with digestive secretions in the stomach.

Clostridium difficile (C. difficile) A bacterium that harbors a toxin that causes an inflamed colon (colitis) and diarrhea. (The ill effects may arise after antibiotics are taken. Previously, and erroneously, these ill effects were thought to be caused by the antibiotic.)

colectomy Surgical removal of all or part of the colon.

colic Pertaining to the colon, or a spasm in an organ accompanied by pain.

colitis Inflammation of the colon (-itis means inflamed).

colon The large intestine, from the end of the ileum (the small intestine) to the rectum. The colon is divided into four parts—the ascending, transverse, descending, and sigmoid (or pelvic) colon—and is responsible for the final phase of digestion and for converting the waste material from foods into solid feces.

colonoscopy An internal examination of the upper portion of the colon with an elongated speculum or an endoscope.

colon polyp An abnormal fleshy growth in the colon. Polyps bleed easily and some types are believed to be susceptible to becoming malignant (cancerous).

constipation Difficult, infrequent, and/or painful bowel movements with hard, dry feces. Sometimes called sluggish bowel.

Crohn's disease A chronic form of inflammatory bowel disease that involves the ileum (the last portion of the small intestine). It is sometimes called regional ileitis or regional enteritis. Symptoms include diarrhea, constipation, vomiting, bloating, abnormally colored stool, abdominal pain, anemia, weight loss, dehydration, fistulas, obstruction of the bowel, and pain around the navel or in the lower-right quadrant of the abdomen.

defecation A bowel movement, the elimination of feces from the colon through the anus.

dehydration An unhealthy loss of fluid from the body; results when fluid output (as from sweat or urine) exceeds fluid intake.

diaphragm The dome-shaped muscle that separates the chest and stomach cavities.

digestion The mechanical and chemical process whereby food is broken down into nutritional components suitable for absorption into the blood and use by individual cells, and waste matter is separated for elimination.

dilation Expansion of an organ or vessel. Also called dilatation.

distention To be uncomfortably swollen with air; an uncomfortable swelling in the intestines.

diverticulitis Inflammation of one or more diverticula in the intestinal tract; may be chronic or acute. Symptoms of the chronic form include worsening constipation, mucus in the stools, and periodic griping abdominal pain. Acute symptoms include inflammation, abscess formation, gangrene, and perforation of the intestinal wall. See also: diverticulum.

diverticulosis The condition of having diverticula without inflammation, pain, or other symptoms (-osis means condition).

diverticulum A pouch, sac, or outpocketing in the wall of an organ or canal. Plural: diverticula.

duodenum The first portion of the small intestine.

dysphagia The inability to swallow or difficulty in swallowing.

dyspepsia See: indigestion.

efferent nerves Nerve fibers that carry signals from the brain and spinal cord to tissue and organs in the body to influence their function. See also: afferent nerves.

elimination diet An eating plan that attempts to identify foods that provoke symptoms by excluding them from a person's diet.

emulsifier A substance that allows incompatible liquids (such as oil and water) to merge into a single solution. In the body, bile produced in the liver emulsifies dietary fats so that they can be absorbed by the blood.

endorphins A group of powerful biochemicals produced naturally in the brain that have morphine-like pain-relieving properties.

endoscope A small, thin, flexible tube with a light and a camera lens used to examine canals and hollow organs, such as the esophagus, stomach, small and large intestines, and the rectum.

endoscopy Examination or treatment facilitated by an endoscope. See also: colonoscopy; enteroscopy; esophogealgastroduodenoscopy (EGD); sigmoidoscopy, sigmoid exam.

enteral tube feeding Administering nutrients by means of a tube passed into the stomach via the nasal passage. Used with patients who are unable or unwilling to chew or swallow food.

enteric Related to the small intestine (enter- means small intestine).

enteric nervous system The portion of the nervous system dedicated to regulating digestive processes.

enteritis Inflammation of the small intestine.

enterocolitis A serious medical condition in which both the small and large intestines are inflamed. Symptoms include fever, sluggishness, abdominal swelling, nausea, diarrhea, vomiting, and rectal bleeding.

enteroscopy Examination of the small intestine with an endoscope.

epithelium The surface tissue on the inner and outer layers of the organs in the digestive tract.

eructation See: belching.

esophagea Pertaining to the esophagus.

esophageal spasm A severe, usually short-lived, cramplike pain under the breastbone, produced by the esophagus.

esophagitis Inflammation of the esophagus.

esophagus The muscular canal that carries food and liquids from the mouth to the stomach.

esophogealgastroduodenoscopy (EGD) Examination of the esophagus, stomach, and duodenum with an endoscope. Also called gastroscopy, upper endoscopy. See also*:* upper GI series.

fecalith A hard mass (concretion) of feces.

fiber Also called roughage, fiber consists of the components of plant foods that resist digestion and add bulk to feces by absorbing water while passing through the colon. Fibrous foods include whole grains, bran flakes, beans, fruits, leafy vegetables, root vegetables and their skins, and prunes. (Prunes also contain a natural laxative called diphenylisatin.)

fistula A tubelike passage that develops between two organs, vessels, or cavities that are not normally connected. May be congenital or result from illness, injury, or inflammation. A fistula may open to the outside of the body.

flatus Expulsion of gas through a body orifice, especially the anus, commonly called farting.

gallbladder A pear-shaped sac under the liver that stores and concentrates bile, and secretes it into the small intestine.

gastric Pertaining to the stomach. (The prefix gastro- means stomach.)

gastric juices A mixture of pepsin, hydrochloric acid, mucin, and small quantities of other biochemicals secreted by the gastric glands in the stomach to promote digestion.

gastritis Inflammation of the stomach lining.

gastroenteritis Inflammation of the stomach and small intestine.

gastroenterologist A doctor who specializes in disorders of the stomach and intestines.

gastroenterology The medical specialty concerned with the structure and function of the stomach, intestines, and related structures (primarily the esophagus, liver, gallbladder, and pancreas).

gastrointestinal (GI) tract See: alimentary canal.

gastroparesis A delay before food is emptied into the small intestine from the stomach. It often occurs in patients receiving parenteral nutrition (intravenous feeding). See also: total parenteral nutrition.

gastroscopy See: esophogealgastroduodenoscopy.

gastrostomy (g-tube) A surgically created fistula that allows a tube to pass from outside the body into the stomach for enteral tube feeding.

giardiasis An infection of the intestinal tract by the parasite *Giardia lamblia*. Symptoms include fever, cramps, diarrhea, greasy stools, flatulence, nausea, vomiting, weakness, anorexia, weight loss, abdominal distention, and belching.

glucose The most important carbohydrate for metabolism. Glucose occurs naturally in some foods and also is formed during digestion.

gluten A protein found in wheat and other grains. See also: celiac disease.

gluten intolerance See: celiac disease.

gut The bowel or intestines.

h2 (histamine2) receptor blocker Medicines that reduce the amount of stomach acid produced by preventing receptor cells from being stimulated by histamine. (Naturally occurring histamine stimulates the secretion of stomach acid as a normal process of digestion.)

Helicobacter pylori (H. pylori) A bacterium that causes some peptic ulcers.

hemorrhoid A mass of dilated veins around the rectum and anus; may protrude externally or internally. Also called piles. Symptoms include burning, itching, localized pain, and straining to produce a bowel movement.

hepatic Pertaining to the liver.

hepatic flexure syndrome Pain localized around the bend (flexure) of the colon under the liver (the upper-right side of the abdomen) resulting from gas or air trapped in the bend. See also: splenic flexure syndrome.

hiatal hernia An opening in the diaphragm that allows the upper portion of the stomach to protrude into the chest.

hydrogen breath test Used to determine lactose intolerance, this test measures the amount of hydrogen in exhaled air.

hyperalgesia Extreme sensitivity to pain.

hypoglycemia Abnormally low levels of glucose in the blood. Symptoms include headache, rapid heart rate, sweating, nausea, mental confusion, irritability, and feeling faint.

ileostomy A surgically created opening (stoma) in the stomach that allows a portion of the ileum to lead outside the body so that fecal matter can drain into a bag worn on the abdomen.

ileum The lower portion of the small intestine.

imperforate anus A birth defect in which the anus fails to develop. (Imperforate means without an opening; the condition is corrected surgically.)

indigestion The incomplete or imperfect digestion of food. Also called dyspepsia. May result from eating too much or too fast, or from disagreeable foods. Symptoms include pain, nausea, vomiting, heartburn and acid regurgitation, gas and belching. See also: celiac disease, lactose intolerance.

inflammatory bowel disease (IBD) A disease that involves the intestinal tract and require medical intervention. See: Crohn's disease, ulcerative colitis.

insulin A hormone secreted by the pancreas, essential for the metabolism of blood sugar and the maintenance of proper blood sugar levels.

intestinal anastomosis The rejoining of two portions of the bowel.

intestinal angina Abdominal pain, usually after eating, caused by decreased blood flow (ischemia) to the intestines. Also called intestinal ischemia , ischemic colitis.

intestinal ischemia See: intestinal angina.

ischemic colitis *See:* intestinal angina.

jejunostomy (j-tube) Surgical opening of the jejunum (second portion of the small intestine) to allow insertion of a tube for enteral tube feeding.

jejunum The second portion of the small intestine.

lactase The enzyme responsible for the digestion of milk sugar (lactose). Deficient in people with lactose intolerance.

lactose intolerance The inability to digest milk sugar (lactose). Symptoms include abdominal bloating, cramping, and diarrhea.

laparotomy The surgical opening of the stomach (-tomy means incision).

laxative A medicine that facilitates evacuation of the bowels. Also called cathartic, purgative.

lipase A digestive enzyme that breaks down fats.

lower esophageal sphincter The one-way valve between the esophagus and the stomach that, when functioning normally, prevents food and stomach secretions from regurgitating into the esophagus.

lower GI series See: barium enema.

mast cell A large tissue cell important to immune system reactions.

mast cell degranulation The release from the mast cell of granules, small sacs, filled with biochemicals, such as histamine and prostaglandins, that digest pathogens and activate other cells to fight infection.

nasogastric tube (ng-tube) A method of enteral tube feeding in which a tube is passed through the nasal passages to the stomach.

neurotransmitter Chemicals involved in sending messages in the nervous system.

nonulcer dyspepsia Abdominal pain similar to that produced by an ulcer, without an ulcer being present.

palpitation An unusually rapid, strong, or irregular heartbeat.

pancreas A gland that secretes enzymes that affect all classes of foods, and the hormones insulin and glucagon that help to regulate carbohydrate metabolism.

parasympathetic nervous system The branch of the autonomic nervous system that creates calming actions such as decreased heart rate, lower blood pressure, increased gastrointestinal activity. The primary neurotransmitter is acetylcholine. See also: autonomic nervous system, sympathetic nervous system.

peristalsis The wavelike movement of the alimentary canal that moves food along the tubes.

postprandial After meals.

probiotics Beneficial bacteria that establish and maintain normal bowel flora or microorganisms, often prescribed after a course of antibiotics.

proctalgia fugax Severe pain resulting from spasms of the rectal muscles.

prokinetic Describes medications that stimulate gastrointestinal activity and the propulsion of chyme along the alimentary canal.

protease An enzyme that breaks protein into amino acids.

proton pump inhibitor (PPI) Medication that inhibits the secretion of stomach acid.

purgative See: laxative.

radioallergosorbent test (RAST) A blood test used to identify substances that cause an allergic reaction.

rectum The lower end of the colon, leading to the anus. Feces are stored here until elimination.

resection, intestinal Surgical removal of a portion of the intestines due to disease.

rheumatologist A doctor who specializes in joint and muscle pain.

Rome II criteria A set of criteria, established in 1999, used to determine a diagnosis of irritable bowel syndrome.

serotonin (5-hydroxytryptamine, 5-HT) A neurotransmitter and vasoconstrictor that plays an important role in intestinal motility, nausea and vomiting, sleep-wake cycles, and depression.

sigmoidoscopy, sigmoid exam Examination of the rectum and the lowest portion of the colon (the sigmoid) with an endoscope.

sitz bath A warm-water, sometimes medicated, bath used to treat some conditions of the rectum or vagina.

small intestine Divided into three parts—the duodenum, jejunum, and ileum—the small intestine is the primary site where food is separated (digested) into nutritive and waste elements and where the absorption of nutrients into the bloodstream occurs.

somatization Expressing a mental condition as a disturbed bodily function; using physical symptoms for conscious or unconscious gain.

spastic colon A synonym for irritable bowel syndrome, no longer in general use.

sphincter A ring of muscle surrounding an orifice that opens and closes it.

splenic flexure syndrome Pain localized around the bend (flexure) of the colon under the spleen (the upper left side of the abdomen) resulting from gas or air trapped in the bend. See also: hepatic flexure syndrome.

stool specimen A small sample of feces collected after elimination and submitted to a laboratory for analysis.

stricture An abnormal narrowing of a body opening.

sympathetic nervous system The branch of the autonomic nervous system concerned with "fight or flight" responses and reactions to fright, such as increased heart rate and blood pressure, depression or cessation of gastrointestinal activity, dilated pupils, and the erection of hairs and gooseflesh. The primary neurotransmitter is norepinephrine. See also: autonomic nervous system, parasympathetic nervous system.

syndrome A group of signs and symptoms that characterize a particular disease or disorder.

total parenteral nutrition Intravenous feeding of patients who are unable to receive adequate nutrition by mouth. See also: gastroparesis.

tricyclic antidepressants (TCA) Medications used to treat depression. In lower doses, they can help to relieve the abdominal pain associated with irritable bowel syndrome.

ulcer A lesion in the skin or mucous membranes with pain, inflammation, necrosis (death of cells, tissues, or organs), and tissue shedding.

ulcer, duodedenal An ulcer in the duodenum.

ulcer, esophageal An ulcer in the esophagus.

ulcer, gastric An ulcer in the stomach .

ulcer, peptic A sore in the lining of the esophagus, stomach, or duodenum, usually caused by a bacteria, *Helicobacter pylori.*

ulcerative colitis A form of inflammatory bowel disease that causes sores (ulcers) and inflammation in the lining of the colon and rectum. Symptoms include severe diarrhea, bloody diarrhea, abdominal pain, and weight loss.

ultrasound A diagnostic test that uses sound waves to outline the shapes of organs and tissues in the body.

upper endoscopy See: esophogealgastroduodenoscopy.

upper GI series X-ray examination of the esophagus, stomach, and duodenum. To facilitate the X-ray, the patient first drinks a solution of barium sulfate that will coat the esophagus and organs to make them more visible. See also: barium enema, esophogealgastroduodenoscopy.

villi Fingerlike projections inside the small intestine that help to absorb nutrients.

Index

A

abuse, 20, 126
acid reflux disorder. *See* gastroesophageal reflux disease (GERD)
acupuncture, 91, 188–189
adrenaline, 156–157
Advil, 86
alcohol, 13, 67, 88, 108–109
  sugar, 103
allergies, 186
  food, 10, 21, 66, 107
aloe, 184
Alternative Medicine Foundation, 148
Ambien, 79
American Academy of Family Physicians, 144
American Association of Sex Educators, Counselors, and Therapists, 168
American Board of Medical Specialties, 146
American College for the Advancement of Medicine, 192
American College of Gastroenterology, 145
American Council on Science and Health, 192
American Dietetic Association, 50, 116
American Gastroenterological Association, 143, 146
American Holistic Health Organization, 148
American Medical Association, 146
American Pain Foundation, 65, 82
American Psychotherapy & Medical Hypnosis Association, 187
American Society of Clinical Hypnosis, 187
anorexia, 14
antibiotics, 20, 21, 88
anticholinergics, 74, 75
antidepressants, 86, 91
  SSRIs, 73
  tricyclic, 72, 73, 88, 214
antidiarrheals, 74, 75
antispasmodics, 74, 75, 134
anxiety, 167
arthritis, 160
aspartame, 67
aspirin, 13

B

bacteria, 13, 20, 34, 86
  in colon, 32
  digestion and, 32
  overgrowth, 21
  probiotics and, 70–71
"bathroom anxiety," 127
Benson, Herbert, 182
Bentylol/Bentyl, 75
betablockers, 91
biofeedback, 91, 93, 180–181
  pain control and, 180
biopsies, 13, 14
birth control pills, 119
bloating, 9, 15, 18, 118, 124
  reasons for, 38–39
blood
  electrolytes, 10
  in stool, 9, 14
  tests, 10
blood pressure, 156–157, 160, 182
books
  After Any Diagnosis: How to Take Action Against Your Illness Using the Best and Most Current Medical Information, 154
  American Dietetic Association Complete Food and Nutrition Guide, 116
  On Being Ill, 206
  Beyond the Relaxation Response: How

to Harness the Healing Power of Your Personal Beliefs, 192
The Chronic Illness Workbook, 172, 206
The Chronic Pain Solution, 82
Conquering Chronic Fatigue: Answers to America's Most Misunderstood Epidemic, 94
On Death and Dying, 206
Digestive Wellness, 128
Eating and Digestion (Body Systems), 138
The First Year—IBS (Irritable Bowel Syndrome): An Essential Guide for the Newly Diagnosed, 26, 138
The Good Gut Guide: Help for IBS, Ulcerative Colitis, Crohn's Disease, Diverticulitis, and Food Allergies, 40
Gut Wisdom: Understanding and Improving Your Digestive Health, 26, 40, 206
Heal Your Headache: The 1-2-3 Program for Taking Charge of Your Pain, 94
IBS: A Doctor's Plan for Chronic Digestive Troubles: The Definitive Guide to Prevention and Relief, 26, 82
IBS Breakthrough: Healing Irritable Bowel Syndrome for Good with Chinese Medicine, 192
Illness as Metaphor, 206
Indigestion: Living Better with Upper Intestinal Problems from Heartburn to Ulcers and Gallstones, 26
Instant Relief: Tell Me Where It Hurts and I'll Tell You What to Do, 172
The Interstitial Cystitis Survival Guide: Your Guide to the Latest Treatment Options and Coping Strategies, 94
The Irritable Bowel Syndrome & Gastrointestinal Solutions Handbook, 128
The Irritable Bowel Syndrome Sourcebook, 26
Listen to Your Gut, 82
Managing Stress: Principles and Strategies for Health and Wellbeing, 172
Mind, Stress, Emotions: The New Science of Mood, 172
Recrafting a Life: Solutions for Chronic Pain and Illness, 206
The Relaxation & Stress Reduction Workbook, 172
Relief from IBS, 26, 82
The Second Brain: A Groundbreaking New Understanding of Nervous Disorders of the Stomach and Intestines, 82
The Sensitive Gut, 40
Stomachaches (My Health), 138
Tell Me What to Eat If I Have Irritable Bowel Syndrome, 116
Understanding Irritable Bowel Syndrome, 26, 40
A Victim No More: Overcoming Irritable Bowel Syndrome, 26
What You Really Need to Know About Irritable Bowel Syndrome, 128
Your Digestive System (How Your Body Works), 138
bowel movements
changes in, 15, 36
exercise and, 114
frequency of, 8, 9
incomplete, 18
menstruation and, 118
pain with, 9

straining during, 18
brain/gut connection, 72–73
breathing
deep, 166, 178, 179

C

caffeine, 13, 39, 67, 88, 134
calcium channel blockers, 76
cancer
colorectal, 14–15, 107
ovarian, 15
CAT scan, 11
Celexa, 73
celiac disease, 10, 12, 14, 22, 107, 132, 208
chemotherapy, 21
chewing food, 28
children and irritable bowel syndrome, 130–137
counseling and, 135
diagnosis, 130–131, 132–133
gender and, 133
guided imagery therapy and, 136
stress in, 136–137
tests, 14, 22, 132
treatment planning, 134–135
Chinese medicine, 185
cholecystokinin receptor antagonists, 76
cholesterol, 112, 160
chronic fatigue syndrome, 86–87, 126
chronic pelvic pain syndrome, 92–93
chyme, 30
colitis, 208
enterocolitis, 210
ischemic, 74, 120
symptoms, 14
ulcerative, 14, 215
colon
bacteria in, 32
cancer, 14–15
Crohn's disease, 14
diverticulitis and, 14
diverticulosis and, 14
sigmoid, 14
ulcerative colitis, 14
colonic transit time, 32, 34, 120
fiber and, 35
colonoscopy, 11, 14, 107, 209
Complementary and Alternative Healing University, 192
condiments, 102
constipation, 8, 15, 18, 21, 69, 70, 209
aloe for, 184
chronic, 36
with diarrhea, 36
fiber and, 36, 37
reasons for, 36–37
recurrent, 9
serotonin and, 120
cortisol, 160, 182
cramps
abdominal, 18
stomach, 8
Crohn's disease, 14, 38, 209

D

dairy products, 67, 71, 102
Dalmane, 79
depression, 8, 72–73, 86, 87, 92, 109, 126, 169
Desyrel, 79
dextrin, 103
diagnosis, 10–11, 16–17
diarrhea, 8, 14, 15, 21, 70
acute, 35
colonic transit time and, 34
constipation with, 36
diet and, 35
over-the-counter medications, 35
reasons for, 34–35
recurrent, 9
stress and, 34

diet, 96–113
beverages, 97
BRAT, 35
childhood, 134
core, 66
elimination, 66–67, 209
fiber in, 14, 100–101
low-fat, 104–105
migraine and, 90
small meals, 97
triggers, 67
dietitians, 50–51, 107
digestion, 21, 28, 29, 209
alcohol and, 108
bacteria and, 20, 32
colonic transit time in, 32
fiber and, 100
gas and, 38–39
hormones and, 118
mechanics of, 30–31
peristalsis in, 28, 32, 33
serotonin and, 73
Directory of Health Organizations Online, 177
diuretics, 20
diverticulitis, 14, 209
diverticulosis, 14
Donnatal, 75
dopamine, 72
Doral, 79
duodenum, 30
dysregulation spectrum syndrome, 87

E

Edwards, Lawrence, 182
Elavil, 73, 79
Elmiron, 88
employment, stress and, 170–171
endometriosis, 92
endorphins, 114, 122, 210
enzymes, 70, 102, 106
erythrocyte sedimentation rate, 10
estrogen, 118, 119, 122, 126
exercise, 114–115
stress and, 166

F

fatigue, 8, 9, 85
chronic, 86–87
fats, 104–105
FDA. *See* Food and Drug Administration
fedotozine, 76
fever, 9, 86, 87
fiber, 14, 35, 36, 100–101, 210
for children, 134
nonsoluble, 37, 100, 101
requirements, 101
soluble, 37, 100, 101
sources, 37, 100, 101, 134
supplements, 68–69
fibromyalgia, 84–85, 126
flatulence, 9, 14, 18, 68, 101, 124
food
allergies, 10, 21, 66, 107
avoidance, 102
beverages, 97
eating right, 112–113
fundamentals, 96–97
intolerances, 106–107
journals, 98–99
labels, 110–111
portion control, 113
postmeal activity, 97
probiotic, 70–71
spices, 97
temperature, 97
triggers, 67
Food and Drug Administration (FDA), 74, 105, 110, 184
food poisoning, 70
friendships, 55, 165

fructose intolerance, 102–103
fruit, 67, 102, 107, 112

G

gas, 38–39
gastroenteritis, 86, 211
gastroenterologists, 44, 46–47, 211
gastroesophageal reflux disease
(GERD), 12–13, 28, 184, 207
gender
children and irritable bowel
syndrome, 133
chronic fatigue syndrome and, 86
irritable bowel syndrome and, 22
stress and, 156–157
GERD. *See* gastroesophageal
reflux disease
Giardia, 13
GI series tests, 11, 207, 215
glucose, 103, 156–157, 211
gluten intolerance, 10, 21, 66, 211
grains, 112
grapefruit seed extract, 185
guided imagery therapy, 136, 178

H

Halcion, 79
headaches, 85, 86, 133
migraine, 87, 89, 90–91
tension, 91
Health Insurance Portability and
Accountability Act, 45
health team, 42–61
advocate, 54, 205
appointments with, 58
certifications for, 52–53
dietitian, 50–51, 107
doctors, 146–147, 199
gasteroenterologist, 44, 46–47
pharmacist, 48–49
primary care doctor, 43, 44, 45
therapist, 52–53
heartburn, 12, 18, 28
herbal treatment, 184–185
aloe, 184
Chinese medicine, 185
grapefruit seed extract, 185
peppermint oil, 184
primrose oil, 185
psyllium, 185
hiatal hernia, 13, 212
hormones, 72, 114, 118, 122, 124, 160,
188
Hyams, Jeffrey, 134
hypnotherapy, 186–187

I

ileum, 14, 30
immune system, 160, 188
incontinence, 18
infection, 14, 22, 132
bacterial, 20, 34
urinary tract, 88
viral, 20, 34
inflammatory bowel disease, 14, 22, 132
insurance, 59, 171
Intelihealth, 145
International Foundation for Functional
Gastrointestinal Disorders, 142
Internet, 140–153. *See also* Web sites
advertising on, 140
evaluating Web sites on, 140–141
finding support groups, 60–61,
150–151
newsgroups, 152–153
search tips, 143
support groups, 150–151
using, 141
interstitial cystitis, 88–89
intestines
large, 32, 33
small, 31

irritable bowel syndrome
acceptance stage, 197
age and, 22, 127
anger over, 197
brain/gut connection, 72–73
causes, 20–21
children and, 130–137
constipation-predominant, 18, 36–37, 74, 114
defining, 161
denial stage, 196
diagnosing, 10–11
diarrhea-predominant, 18, 30, 34–35, 74, 120
diet and, 50, 66–67
digestion and, 28–29
exercise and, 114–115
fat and, 104–105
friends and, 55, 165
as functional disorder, 16
gender and, 22, 118–127
health team for, 42–61
hormones and, 118–119
living with, 194–205
menstruation and, 118–119
mind/body issues, 175
nutrition and, 96–113
pain-predominant, 18
positive attitudes and, 200–201
pregnancy and, 124
relationships and, 168–169
similar/overlapping conditions, 12–15, 84–93
sleep and, 78–79
stages of adjustment to, 196–197
symptoms, 8, 9
talking about, 202–203
testing for, 10–11
treatment, 63–82
triggers, 21, 24, 67, 80
types of, 18–19
waxing and waning of, 23
Irritable Bowel Syndrome Association, 143

J

jejunum, 30, 30
Journal of the American Medical Association, 144
journals, 24–25
food, 98–99
recording changes, 56–57

K

kappa opioids, 122
Kübler-Ross, Elisabeth, 196

L

labels, food, 110–111
Lactaid, 71
lactose intolerance, 10, 21, 34, 66, 71, 106, 132, 212
laxatives, 37, 68–69, 213
Levbid/Levsin, 75
Lexapro, 73
Lomotil, 75
Lotronex, 74, 75, 120–121, 125
Luvox, 73
lymph nodes, 86

M

Mayo Clinic, 145
meats, processed, 67, 102
medications
antacids, 68
antibiotic, 20, 21, 88
anticholinergic, 74, 75
antidepressant, 72–73, 86, 88, 91, 214
vantidiarrheal, 68, 74, 75
vantigas, 68
antihistamine, 78
anti-inflammatory, 88

antispasmodic, 19, 74, 75, 134
betablockers, 91
buying online, 49
diarrheal, 35
diuretics, 20
gender and, 120–121
laxatives, 19, 37
nonsteroidal anti-inflammatory, 86
over-the-counter, 8, 35, 48, 68–69, 184
during pregnancy, 125
probiotics, 35
serotonin receptor agonists, 75
side effects, 73, 74, 75, 78
sleep, 78–79
meditation, 182–183
techniques, 182, 183
Medline Plus, 144
menopause, 119
menstruation, 118–119
migraine
abdominal, 90
diet and, 90
headaches, 89, 90–91
triggers, 90
monosodium glutamate, 67
Motrin, 86
mucus, 18
muscarinic receptor antagonists, 76

N

National Association of Cognitive-Behavioral Therapists, 81
National Certification Commission for Acupuncture and Oriental Medicine, 189
National Institute of Diabetes & Digestive & Kidney Diseases, 144
National Institutes of Health, 180, 188
National Center for Complementary and Alternative Medicine, 148, 176, 177, 192
National Mental Health Association, 147
National Migraine Association, 94
National Qigong Association, 191
National Women's Health Resource Center, 145
nausea, 8, 14, 18, 91, 133
nervous system
autonomic, 182, 207
central, 72
dysregulation spectrum syndrome and, 87
enteric, 72, 210
parasympathetic, 213
sympathetic, 214
newsgroups, 152–153
nitric oxide, 70
nonsteroidal anti-inflammatories, 86
noradrenalin, 90
norepinephrine, 73, 156–157
Norpramin, 73
nutrition, 96–113
Daily Reference Values and, 111
fat and, 104–105
fiber, 14, 35, 36, 37, 100–101
fructose in, 102–103
total parenteral, 214
nutritionists, 50–51
nuts, 67

O

obesity, 160
octreotide, 76

P

pain
abdominal, 9, 14, 16, 21, 118, 120, 131
blocking, 65, 89
childhood, 130
chronic, 182
chronic pelvic, 92–93

control of, 180–181, 182, 186
coping with, 64–65
factors, 65
joint, 85
menstrual, 87
onset factors, 65
rectal, 120
recurrent, 131
sensitivity to, 74, 84
sexual, 92, 123
stomach, 70, 130
urinary, 88
women and, 122–123
Pain Net, Inc., 147
parasites, 13
Paxil, 73
peppermint oil, 184–185
peristalsis, 28, 32, 33, 213
pharmacists, 48–49
phenylethamines, 76
physical therapy, 93
polyps, 14–15
posttraumatic stress disorder, 126
pregnancy, 124–125, 160
premenstrual syndrome, 118
primrose oil, 185
Pro-Banthine, 75
probiotics, 35, 64, 70–71, 213
choosing, 71
progesterone, 118, 119, 126
Prosom, 79
prostaglandin, 118
Prozac, 73
psychotherapy, 23, 52–53, 81
cognitive-behavioral, 80, 81
psyllium, 185

Q

qigong, 191
Quack Watch, 149
Questran, 75

R

recurrent abdominal pain syndrome, 131
relaxation, 166–167
meditation and, 182
muscle, 178
progressive, 178
remedies. *See* medications
resources. *See* books; Web sites
restless legs syndrome, 87
Restoril, 79
Rome II Diagnostic Criteria, 16–17, 214
roughage. *See* fiber

S

serotonin, 72, 73, 78, 84, 90, 120, 214
agonists, 74
sexual intercourse, 92, 123
sigmoidoscopy, 11, 214
Sinequan, 73, 79
sleep, 78–79
disturbance, 85, 87
life style and, 78
smoking, 88
Sonata, 79
sorbitol, 102, 103, 134
spices, 97
stevia, 103
stool
abnormal passage, 9
blood in, 9
hard, 18
incontinence, 18
loose, 18
mucus in, 18
tests, 11
stress, 20, 23, 52, 114, 156–171
attitude adjustment and, 162
childhood, 136–137
chronic, 158–159, 166–167
coping with, 137, 158–159, 162–163
deep breathing and, 166, 178

defining, 156–157
diarrhea and, 34
exercise and, 166
"fight-or-flight," 156
gender and, 156–157
inventory of, 164–165
job-related, 170–171
long-term, 158–159
management, 178–179
negative coping responses to, 159
physical ailments from, 160–161
reduction, 64, 72, 88
response to, 156–157
role of, 64
short-term, 156–157
travel and, 163
sucrose, 102
sugars, 102–103, 113
support groups, 60–61, 150–151
swallowing, 28
symptoms
chronic fatigue syndrome, 87
chronic pelvic pain syndrome, 93
colitis, 14
depression, 86
fibromyalgia, 85
interstitial cystitis syndrome, 89
irritable bowel syndrome, 8, 9

T

tai chi, 191
telecommuting, 170
tests, 10–11
blood, 10, 14, 22, 132
body imaging, 11
CAT scan, 11
celiac sprue, 10
colonic transit time, 11
colonoscopy, 11, 107
endoscopy, 11, 13
erythrocyte sedimentation rate, 10
GI series, 11, 207, 215
hydrogen, 103
lactose intolerance, 10
pelvic, 11
physical examinations, 11
sigmoidoscopy, 11
stool, 11
therapy, 174–191
acupuncture, 188–189
biofeedback, 91, 93, 180–181
complementary, 174–191
herbal, 184–185
hypnotherapy, 186–187
meditation, 182–183
psychotherapy, 23, 52–53, 81
qigong, 191
tai chi, 191
vitamins and, 184–185
yoga, 190–191
time management, 162
Tofranil, 73
transcutaneous electrical nerve stimulation (TENS), 89, 93
treatment, 63–82
alternative, 174–191
children, 134–135
with complementary therapies, 174–191
herbal/botanical, 184–185
plans, 64–65, 134–135

U

ulcers, 160, 214
duodedenal, 215
esophageal, 215
gastric, 215
peptic, 13, 215

V

vegetables, 67, 102, 107, 112
virus, 34, 86

vitamins, 184–185
vomiting, 8
vulvar vestibulitis, 92

W

water, 97
Web sites
evaluating, 140–141
www.aafp.org, 144
www.aap.org, 138
www.aapb.org, 181
www.aasect.org, 168
www.abms.org, 146
www.aboutibs.org, 142
www.aboutkidsgi.org, 138, 142
www.acam.org, 192
www.acg.gi.org, 145
www.acsh.org, 192
www.ahha.org, 148
www.alternativehealing.org, 192
www.ama_assn.org, 146
www.amfoundation.org, 148
www.apmha.com, 187
www.asch.net, 187
www.bcia.org, 181
www.bestdoctors.com, 147
www.cfids.org, 94
www.eatright.org, 62, 116
www.faqs.org, 152
www.fibrohugs.com, 94
www.gastro.org, 62, 143, 146
www.goaskalice.columbia.edu, 145
www.groups.yahoo.com, 151
www.webring.com/hub?ring=ibs, 26
www.healthywomen.org, 145
www.ibis-australia.org, 40
www.ibsassociation.org, 143
www.ibsgroup.org, 26, 40, 150
www.ibshealth.com, 128
www.ic-network.com, 94
www.iffgd.org, 62
www.intelihealth.com, 145
www.ivillage.com, 151
www.jama.ama-assn.org, 144
www.mayoclinic.com, 145
www.med.unc.edu/wrkunits/2depts/medicine/fgidc/welcome.htm, 40
www.migraines.org, 94
www.nacbt.org, 81, 82
www.nccam.nih.gov, 148, 192
www.niddk.nih.gov, 40, 144
www.nlm.nih.gov, 177
www.nlm.nih.gov/medlineplus/irritablebowelsyndrome.html, 128, 144
www.nmha.org, 62, 147
www.painnet.com, 147
www.panix.com/ibs, 26
www.pelvicpain.org, 94
www.quackwatch.org, 149
www.romecriteria.org, 26
www.socialworkers.org, 62
www.theacpa.org, 82
www.thehealthresource.com, 154
www.wholehealthmd.com, 128
weight loss, 8, 9, 14, 15, 133
wheat products, 67
women. *See also* gender
irritable bowel syndrome and, 118–127
medications and, 120–121
oral contraceptives, 119
pain and, 122–123
premenstrual syndrome and, 118
stress and, 156–157

Y

yoga, 190–191
Yunus, Muhammad, 87

Z

Zelnorm, 74, 75, 120–121, 125
Zoloft, 73